Stillness and Concentration

Other books by Elisabeth Lukas

Meaning and Suffering

The Therapist and the Soul

In the series
Viktor Frankl's Living Logotherapy:

Understanding *Man's Search for Meaning*:
Reflections on Viktor Frankl's Logotherapy

A Unique Approach to Family Counseling:
Logotherapy, Crisis, and Youth

Stillness and Concentration:
Logotherapy Applied to Tinnitus and Chronic Illness

Meaningful Living:
Introduction to Logotherapy Theory and Practice

Stillness and Concentration

Logotherapy Applied to Tinnitus and Chronic Illness

Elisabeth Lukas

Translated by Manfred Hillmann and John de Paor

Part B translated by
Joseph Fabry, Bianca Hirsch, Howard Smith, and James O'Meara

Edited by Charles McLafferty, Jr.

Book 3: *Viktor Frankl's Living Logotherapy* series

Purpose **R**esearch

Charlottesville, Virginia

Published by Purpose Research, llc, Box 5032, Charlottesville, Virginia 22905 USA
http://PurposeResearch.com charles@purposeresearch.com
Back cover photograph © 2014 Charles McLafferty, Jr.
Cover design, layout, and typesetting by Purpose Research

The following chapters (translated by Joseph Fabry) are reprinted gratefully from *The International Forum for Logotherapy*: 19: "Meaning and goals in the chronically ill"; 20: "The 'birthmarks' of paradoxical intention": 21: "A validation of logotherapy"; 22: "Counseling tactics and personality structure"; 23: "Logotherapy on hysteria"; 24: "The meaning of logotherapy for clinical psychology." Chapter 19 was also published in Lukas, E. (1992). *Psychotherapy with dignity*, (Joseph Fabry, Howard Smith, and James O'Meara, trans.). Published privately by the author.

Poems after Chapters 19-24 are from Lukas, E. (1992). *Meaningful lines: Logophilosophical wisdom* (Hirsch, B. & Fabry, J., trans.). Berkeley: Institute of Logotherapy Press.

This book is published for educational purposes only and is not intended for the diagnosis and/or treatment of medical or mental health disorders. All who need help with any such disorder are encouraged to consult with a qualified logotherapist or helping professional.

For more information about the work of Elisabeth Lukas around the world, please visit the Lukas Archives: http://elisabeth-lukas-archiv.de

For more information about training in logotherapy and existential analysis search for "Viktor Frankl Institute" and "Elisabeth Lukas Archive" on the web.

ISBNs: 978-1-948523-264 (Hardcover)
978-1-948523-06-6 (Paperback)

Library of Congress Control Number: 2019951525

9 8 7 6 5 4 3 2 1

Contents

Foreword

Recently, a news article revealed hidden details of an official photograph of a well-known world leader. Notably, it had been altered subtly to portray him more favorably. His shoulders were broadened, the torso slimmed, the face touched up. Even the index finger on his outstretched hand had been lengthened, presumably to show greater power.

In this media-driven world, images are powerful tools. A photograph can be combined with words to have an impact on viewers—indeed, we have a special word for it: a *meme*. The same picture can be used to impact viewers positively or negatively, depending on the words used and the manipulation of the visual image—e.g., color vs. black and white, crystal clear vs. grainy and muddled, closeup vs. distant.

The manipulation of meaning to influence and even to control our thinking and perception is nothing new; it predates even Gutenberg's printing press. Every society has had "town criers" or "influencers" who had far more connections than the average person and used them for various ends. It is only recently, however, that individuals have determined how to use Facebook, Instagram, Twitter, Snapchat, and YouTube to capture the attention of millions of people at once.

This point was brought home to me when I met a person who has helped to develop an immensely popular board game. It turned out that we had something in common, as we were both heading out to present at conferences. He asked me how large my conference was, and I told him a few hundred. He replied that he didn't "waste his time" with conferences that small, as his "minimum" was five to ten thousand attendees. We talked for a few minutes, and he left me with a stunning admission: "It's all about attention. If we can get them to pay attention to our game for even one more second, that's what it's all about."

And that's the key: *capturing and controlling our attention.* There is so much visual, auditory, and sensory stimulation available to us that it is often hard to know who. we. are. The constant din that surrounds us leaves very little room for an awareness of an inner silence that is always available and ever present. How can we know who we are if there is no place in which to experience that quiet, inner space, that place where we know our true selves?

From a logotherapeutic standpoint, the single factor here for us to consider is our area of freedom. It is this tiny area for which we are responsible. So many things have hijacked our power of attention, our ability to choose our focus. Do we continue to choose to turn our attention to an outrageous tweet from world leaders who—on purpose—evoke righteous indignation in order to distract us from the truth? Do we continue to choose to focus on the horrors and calamities inflicted on the poor and suffering by the Merchants of Illusion? Do we choose to focus on our own shortcomings, on the symptoms of a chronic illness, on the incessant ringing in our ears?[1]

In our tiny area of freedom, we can choose to adopt the stance of what has been called "the Observer" in these moments. We can *observe* the outrageous tweets. We can *observe* the horror presented to us by the news media. We can *observe* our symptoms—yes, they are part of our experience, but they are not who we are. By quietly and dispassionately observing, we preserve our freedom to choose our most meaningful response in each of these cases. Moreover, we have the power to choose the pictures that we hold in our mind's eye—and the words that we use to create our own "mind-memes."

Perhaps we are reaching the point in the development of humanity where our only remaining choice is, indeed, the focus of our attention. In this book, *Stillness and Concentration*, Elisabeth Lukas presents a series of vignettes and stories that help the individual deal with unavoidable suffering. This volume contains that entire book, translated by Manfred Hillmann and John de Paor, followed by a keynote address given by Lukas on meaning

---

1   Of course, it goes without saying that we should do everything possible within reason to ameliorate any symptoms that are bothering us—symptoms of illness require appropriate investigation!

and goals in those with chronic illness. Additional articles address various aspects of a psychotherapy with dignity—an approach that preserves the inherent freedom of those who are being helped.

About this series

Over the years, Lukas has written more than 50 books, which have been translated into 19 languages. She has given keynote addresses and lectures at numerous universities and conferences, including many of the World Congresses of Logotherapy. Her writings have been translated into English for print in books and journals, particularly *The international forum for logotherapy: Journal of search for meaning*. For years, I have wanted to collect these writings in a book form. I am personally grateful for the support of Elisabeth Lukas and the Lukas Archive, as well as others who have given so unselfishly of their time and energy to help move this project forward.

The first book, *Understanding Man's Search for Meaning: Reflection on Viktor Frankl's logotherapy*, is one of four volumes published simultaneously. It contains some of the most insightful and profound expansions of logotherapy into the problems of our time. Many of these chapters are drawn from keynote addresses to World Congresses of Logotherapy. Until now, the English versions have mainly been privately published, though some have appeared in the *The international forum*.

A second volume, *A unique approach to family counseling: Logotherapy, crisis, and youth* focuses on the application of logotherapy in families and relationships. It includes articles from *The international forum*, book chapters, and keynote speeches.

This, the third volume, has already been described: The first part of this book is a translation of *Stillness and concentration: Logotherapy for tinnitus and chronic diseases*. The rest of the book contains articles and presentations that fall broadly under the topic of "psychotherapy with dignity."

A new edition of *Meaningful living: Introduction to logotherapy theory and practice* is the fourth book in the series. Part A contains a revision of the 1984 classic, *Meaningful living: Logotherapeutic guide to health*. Part B adds an article by Elisabeth Lukas and Bianca Hirsch that was originally published in the *Comprehensive handbook of psychotherapy, vol. 3*. Many of the cases summarized in Part B can be found in more detail in the original text of *Meaningful living*, and are cross-referenced throughout. This archival article also documents the history of logotherapy as of 2002.

To the extent possible, these books have been edited for a new generation of logotherapists. Sentences have been restructured whenever possible to use inclusive language (including sex, race, culture, and gender identity) and to minimize labeling (e.g., "person with an addiction disorder" instead of "addict") in accordance with the *Publication Manual of the American Psychological Association* (6th ed). Further, the translation of these concepts from German into English occasionally resulted in difficult-to-understand passages, and these have been revised and even rewritten. If, as a result of this work, meaning has been lost or changed, that is solely my fault, and for that I take full responsibility. Hopefully, the inherent meaning will shine through when English words are inadequate to express it.

It is hoped that these books will serve to kindle interest in the meaning possibilities available to all of us, and in so doing to ignite the flames of meaning among those who sense there is something more to life.

To each reader, no matter at what stage in life, regardless of your setbacks, failures, and fate, there awaits a purpose that only you can fulfill, one for which you were created. It is the discovery of, orientation to, and *action on* this possibility that brings meaning. Even a few minutes a day pursuing this unique life mission will result in a harvest of positive fruits and help you to build a monument of meaning that can never be taken away… in time or in eternity.

Charles McLafferty, Jr.
University of Virginia
June, 2019

Part A

Stillness and Concentration:
Logotherapy Applied to
Tinnitus and Chronic Illness

Introduction: Listening to Silence

A voice with an authority beyond the human resounds within the person; Viktor E. Frankl stated this idea in his *Ten theses about the person*. The particular indications for living contained within this voice will then be worked out by the conscience.

Countless other soul explorers, prophets, and healers from both East and West have announced similar findings in their own words. Their message is that something echoes through the heart of the human person and calls for attention, that a gentle inner voice speaks truth, tells of good and evil, notes what is fitting for human beings, indicates how things should be done with a minimum of error in our daily actions. The human heart somehow finds its way through life's many entanglements, though never with total success, as if listening to a song sung to some lofty primeval music.

One thing is made clear in all such descriptions: This mystical element within us, and resounding through us, can be heard only in stillness. Only when the noise levels of outer industry and inner busyness are scaled down, when wrestling thoughts fall limp, when petty fears are shaken off and peace has settled in, only then will an individual become receptive to any signals coming from the depths of the soul. It is for this reason that all cultures have developed rituals of contemplation, methods of meditation, and forms of prayer whose aim it is to advance these explorations into stillness, this search for some sound of a word from the mystery.

But ours is an extremely noisy world. Wave after wave of traffic noise breaks on our doors. Our work place is filled with pounding. The din of quarrelling pervades the home. And there is hardly need to mention the victorious sounds of the entertainment industry with its endless rhythmical roar in night clubs, homes, cars, shopping malls, and supermarkets. With headphones it has advanced even into the final safe haunts of our personal existence. Zones of quiet are not easily found anymore, and must now be sought out. Silence has become precious for its rarity.

These are the facts: The incidence of physical ear ailments—hearing loss—is on the increase. There are high levels of "nerves" and irritability. We have lost contact spiritually with our "inner voice." Taking all these together, one can speak of our being in a daze and stumbling about, because we have become deaf to the tender tones, the gentle, soft movements of the heart. In the hubbub of excessive noise what can humanly exalt us gets swamped, and all too often what is itself human can become obscured.

But nature has its own ways and means of coping. If things become too hectic it will always come up with an alternative, and it is not always so fussy about the means it will employ. Perhaps the sudden huge rise in tinnitus cases in our day—almost 30% of the population suffers from it occasionally, 10% chronically—can be seen as an example. Tinnitus not only brings with it bad moods, interrupted sleep, and even depression, but it can also bring with it an immense longing for quiet. This is good—not the suffering, but the longing. It will also change somewhat one's consciousness, because of the continuous humming and buzzing sound.

Tinnitus sufferers would gladly run a mile from it, but this is not possible. They must ask themselves: "What would I truly be running from?" From all the superficial rubbish that consumerism keeps insisting that we need, and from the accursed war of illusions that insists on whitewashing this destitution and emptiness... what Frankl termed the *existential vacuum*. But the whitewashing is unable to turn it into any kind of reality that can satisfy. Those surrounded by this inescapable and never-ending din, together with its echo within, soon come to their senses searching out for some refuge of silence, and, as luck would have it, this brings them back, once more, to their own respective center.

From this point of view, tinnitus, like any other serious disability, carries its own challenge and message, which could be put like this: You will have to acquire new hearing, not that of physical ears, but rather of the heart's ears. You must develop what Frankl called your organ of meaning, the *conscience*, which hears the daily and hourly call knocking on your door, the call to a concretely meaningful form of existence. You must *listen for the message*, not simply to the sounds.

Just as music is not merely the juxtaposition of sounds, so your life is not just a series of days and hours. Rather, it is what you make of it, a one-off work of art by a special person, unrepeatable, different, and unlike anything else in this vast universe. Therefore, turn away from the empty sounds to savor with your spiritual ears the reverse side of all noise. Nourish yourself on silence, replenish yourself there, and listen to the messages that are being passed on to you in it, through it.

Whoever arrives at this point and is thus able to understand suffering has discovered that there is some value in it. This change to a meaning-centered life also brings healing. In fact, there are many pains and handicaps, which, when they can be confined to the bodily and psychological level, will perceptibly shrink in significance. The person who is attuned to his or her conscience is quite simply tuned in some octaves higher than the one who is only picking up the noise of the daily invasive din.

This book's purpose is to offer a series of psychological helps from Frankl's treasury of ideas. The reader is invited, through an attentive reading, to "co-hear" what may emerge from the letters and lines. It is hoped that, in this manner, something will so deeply touch those who suffer that the all-pervading backdrop of outer and inner harassment can, for a time, be forgotten. The noise will, of course, still be there, but it will not have power over the sufferer because it is no longer given attention. When something real impinges on one's existence, awareness can be placed on that which is infinitely more important and of more value than this present existence (this applies especially for the sufferers of tinnitus and similar hearing problems); *the better one hears with the heart the less one hears with one's physical ears.* What a wonderful exchange! This similarly applies for any chronic illness: *The more sensitive and open one is to the deeper values the less one is hemmed in by the distress flowing from one's illness.*

Here, then, are the promised helps in the form of a varied mix of philosophical, psychological, and anecdotal examples. They are offered in support of the simple and yet eternally comforting truth that bodily handicaps are, in principal, levers for the advancement and development of our spirits and souls. They will often contribute also to the perfection of our human existence.

CHAPTER ONE

A Fulfilled Life Despite Pain

In each person's heart lies a fundamental wish for a meaningful life. However, this idea is given little attention while everything is going well. But if things go wrong, then questions about life's meaning may rise to the surface. This explains why we seldom have an explicit awareness of the meaning of our own existence worked out in advance.

Often, it is only an extreme situation that brings us face to face with the decision whether ours is to be an embittered "no"—or an unconditional "yes"—to life. Such a choice does not allow for any middle ground. And such a judgement, once made, often endures for a long time.

The story of a couple I know comes to mind. Their seven-year old son fell ill with leukemia. With the help of many transfusions the boy lived for three years. But the important point is that these three years turned out to be a very special time for the family. They counted like 30 years, as the couple assured me, not for their difficulties but because of their intensity.

When he felt strong enough for it, the child was allowed to go to school to be with his classmates. When he was weak, he was carried to the playground to be able to watch the other children playing. A third of the children's room was cleared out to make room for a model railway, and many hours were spent together in assembling it. There were also reading sessions that opened up the boy's mind to the fantasy realms of sagas and fairy tales. A beautiful carved xylophone was acquired, upon which the weak hands of the child sent gentle melodies resounding throughout the house. Was all this meaningless, simply because this young life ended early? His parents emphatically disagreed. Precisely because of the pressure of time, it was absolutely correct. In fact, it was wonderful that the child had these experiences. Of course, the pain of his illness was allowed its full impact, and yet this pain seemed to be of little significance in the face of a deeply fulfilled, happy family.

The individual is able to know human existence as precious—and to say "yes" to it—not because of its length or its lustful pleasures, but rather its content, that to which it is *dedicated*. The word "dedicated" has a somewhat solemn sound, and indeed this is exactly what is intended. That which is dedicated to some cause or some beloved, worthy person has the nature of a gift, because that cause or that loved person are more highly regarded than that which is expended on them. It is similar with our lives in general. If they are to have meaning, they must be spent on some cause or on something worthy of our engagement in a self-transcending way. The experience of fulfillment is intensified through ready, conscious dedication to some task. From such a perspective, effort and pain appear insignificant. That this is possible, even in extreme situations, is clearly proven by this example.

Tips for people with tinnitus and chronic illness

Similarly, you may be in such an extreme situation. Permanent, physical-psychological pain accompanies you all the time. But before you begin to doubt the meaningfulness of your existence, consider this: Beyond the pain, is there something or someone to whom you might wish to dedicate your life? Discovering such a productive purpose will determine your choice, which is full of implications for your future, between a bitterness about your illness which will shatter you, or a rising above it, which can bring you fulfillment.

CHAPTER TWO

No One is Superfluous or Replaceable

B y way of contrast, here is an example of a life bereft of meaning: A woman was referred to me who had jumped from a first-floor window, but she had come out of it with little or no damage. She described to me her act of desperation as follows:

> I thought to myself, that my husband could, if I were once dead, marry a nicer and happier woman, and that my children would breathe again having been freed from the nagging of their mother. I thought, further, that no one would miss me, neither the shop assistants in the local store that I visited daily, nor the mere acquaintances who felt obliged to drop in occasionally to see us. Whether I exist or not makes no difference to the world.

This woman suffered from no illness or chronic physical pain, but rather from a feeling of being worthless. She saw herself as useless and superfluous, and thus virtually as a burden for her family and her neighbors. How does one reply to such a case? There are two theses to consider. This is how I formulate the first one:

Every individual deed that we do is our spiritual "fingerprint," as it were, personal, unique, and one that cannot be replicated by anyone else.

What does this mean? Something wonderful, actually. Nothing that a person does, says, or sets in motion… is identical with that which another person does, says, or sets in motion. Let 10,000 or 100,000 people paint the same landscape and we will end up with 10,000 or 100,000 different paintings. Or let many people perform some mundane task, such as to sweep the street; then we will end up with just as many distinct acts of sweeping the street.

Of course, there will not be big differences between these distinct acts, except the words exchanged among the sweepers, the expressions on their faces, their moods will all differ. Some will help each other; others will shove aside trash for someone else to collect. Some will be happy and show it by whistling a tune; others may be holding back tears of despair. Some will wield their brush carefully, while others work vigorously and with great determination and will. In all things, even with such a mundane task, the original personality, the distinctive and unique self of the person, is expressed.

The patient in the example was wrong in seeing herself as replaceable, as wife, mother, shopper in the local market. Yes, her task, her role could be filled by anyone, but *she—as a person—was irreplaceable*. Her death would mean that her uniqueness would disappear with her from this world, as would her own special range of influence. By way of clarification, I told her about the true story of identical twin brothers who took up similar avocations, and they looked alike even in their external appearance. One of them died of heart failure and left a grieving family. Afterwards, whenever the other brother came on a visit to the house the children took fright and would hide themselves under the bed. They thought this was not an optical illusion but that their dead father had come home—though he was *not their father* in spite of having the same voice, the same beard on the same face. It was not the same person. Without understanding this anthropological phenomenon, the children sensed it and rejected this "substitute."

My patient was amazed that she should be considered irreplaceable. "What is special about me?" she asked.

I confronted her with a mirror: "You see this woman, who on a certain day chose to be the lifelong companion of her husband. The woman who bore your children. This is a woman who makes decisions about things that have the potential of preparing these children for heaven or hell. A woman who can add to or take from the good spirits of her local shopkeeper, her guests or whoever she happens to meet. She can take up her house duties with energy or half-heartedly, she can put on this or that style as she likes, whether to please herself or for others. This is what is special about her that she can at any moment choose anew from any of a thousand possibilities...."

Dumbfounded and overcome, she stared at her reflection. "I never realized that I had the choice," she finally whispered, "or that my choice would matter that much. Perhaps I should look at myself with more consideration after all."

Tips for people with tinnitus and chronic illness

Never forget that you are unique. Crowds of other sick people may suffer the same ringing in the ears and disabilities as you do, but no other person will react just as you do. For it is you—and not the noise in your ears—who makes the choice as to how you deal with yourself and your symptoms, and what differences you will radiate into the world around you. With every choice you make, you leave a spiritual "fingerprint" which carries your personal stamp. Whether special for its quality, for its helplessness, its bravery... whatever it is, the choice is yours.

CHAPTER THREE

Something Important Awaits Each Person

We now come to the second thesis, which runs as follows: *Any and every detail in the life of a person can hold a hidden meaning, which may only be revealed at a later time.*

All that happens in the lives of the creatures of this earth is interconnected and interrelated. No creature can exist without the others. In a similar fashion the building stones of our lives are united with the destinies of other people. If even one of these sustaining stones were to be removed, a whole chain would collapse.

This reminds me of my father, who recounted to me how curious for knowledge he was as a child in the 1920s. He had a special empathy with his language teacher in school, who was able to teach the prescribed languages in such an interesting way that my father loved these classes, and became interested in learning noncompulsory foreign languages as well; in particular, Slavic languages that were not taught in the school. His teacher helped him and invited my father to share in free lunchtime lessons. He also lent him books from his rich library of foreign-language books.

All this was more or less fun and games, a rose by the wayside, plucked by my father, but with no idea of any deeper meaning being sensed. There was no way he could have suspected, as a child, how serious these games would appear 15 years later, when World War II broke out and he was sent to the front as a ordinary soldier. Doubtless, he would have been left behind in some trench, that is to say in a trench-grave, if it were not for the fact that he had been ordered back from the front to a safer place to do some translating because of his linguistic knowledge. An experience in his youth may have saved my father's life and put him in a position to pass life on to me. In this way I owe my existence to some teacher I never met, who in his day was glad to take seriously an inquisitive kid and indulge his thirst for knowledge while thinking nothing about using up his own free time.

Often we have no inkling about meaning, indeed nothing of the meaning of the thorns involved in the picking of roses, and yet every detail of our experience at a particular point in time and a particular place can have a huge importance for us and for those who live around us. From this point of view, the woman mentioned in the last chapter who jumped out of the window was in error because she considered it to be of no importance whether or not she existed. It was not unimportant, because with her untimely death the meaning of many events in her life, which might have later come to fruition, would no longer be possible.

Who could have guaranteed to her then that sometime, somehow, some task might not have presented itself to her, that only one with *her* experience, only she with *that* rose in her hand which she had picked, or someone with *that* scratch *she* had received from the thorns, could deal with? Often we do not know what possibilities result from something that happens to us but it is good to remember that *everything that happens to us contains the potential for meaning.*

Regardless, the story about my father's language teacher inspired this patient to volunteer her help in giving extra coaching in German lessons to foreign students. In this way she came to know Ali, whose Syrian father could not get permission to immigrate and whose German mother had been murdered in Syria. The orphaned and uprooted Ali would really rather have liked to die. How well my patient was able to understand this young man! She vibrated on the same wavelength with his sensibility. She gently established a friendship with the young lad, helped him through his difficulties and integrated him more and more into her own family. As we were concluding our therapeutic sessions I was able to see the youngster briefly. He held on closely to his new foster mother, played with her and teased her.

"Do you now realize what is unique about you?" I asked her, "or should Ali explain it to you?"

"It is not necessary," she replied, pointing with a nod towards the mirror. "I have grasped that something is stored up for each one of us. In the meantime I have come to know"—at this, she gently stroked the lad's untamable hair—"who was waiting for me!"

Tips for people with tinnitus and chronic illness

You do not need to jump out of the window in order to come to the realization that there is something important in store for you. At the moment, perhaps you cannot imagine what that might be. Perhaps you are too busy with the daily struggle to maintain your mental and emotional balance. Or it may not yet have become clear, simply because it is still in the far future. But there is one thing you can correctly assume: Your present precarious health situation is, in some mysterious way, a meaningful prerequisite for what is waiting for you out there.

CHAPTER FOUR

Yes, Wonders Do Still Happen!

What is it that gives human beings strength in their time of need? This is an exciting question. I have presented the stories of a married couple and a woman where both have drawn strength through a selfless dedication towards a child. Apart from this, the parallel between the two cases does not go any further; in the first case, the child was dying while in the second, the child began to bloom again. Let us reflect on this. Is it not worth noticing that both the couple and the woman gained strength through their commitment and retained it, though the outcome of their concern was from the start totally uncertain, and as things turned out, totally different.

Psychotherapists—precisely in Frankl's understanding—know about this phenomenon. In practice, the success or outcome of an action is irrelevant. The *act of choosing and the engagement* in themselves produce an elixir and, together with the art of healing, give one the hope of being an unbeatable team.

Perhaps "hope" should be expressed as "belief in miracles" even if that expression is not well accepted; in its purist form, hope is totally at odds with reason. True hope does not hone in on any earthly "happy ending." Rather, it spins a gentle thread that stretches further, into the transcendent dimension, where success is spelled differently than it is in our human—all-too-human—sphere.

This is precisely the way the ground is made ready for the miracle. In hoping against all reason, a crack is often opened wide to receive the dewdrops of transcendence falling on our lot that retroactively bless our commitment. Otto-Heinrich Kühner illustrated this with a story, which took place in the United States:

> Bill, a young man, took Bob, who was blind, for a walk. In the course of the walk, Bob told him the following story: Earlier in life, he had been a pilot and had once flown a plane from Miami to Pernambuco, Brazil. Some explosives were concealed in the luggage of one of the passengers by her husband, in the hope that he would collect her life insurance on her death. Bob described the resulting catastrophe:

> A storm had put us off course, far out over the Atlantic. Then I heard the explosion and knew immediately what it was.... We went into a spin and crashed into the sea. There had been 23 on board, passengers and crew. Six of us were still alive. I could no longer see, because splinters had embedded in my eyes. Then a piece of the plane was floating by and we latched on to it. After four hours, two of the survivors slid under and drowned. They had simply lost their strength. We were to spend the whole night in this state....

> One of the remaining four, Mr. Bernardes, had strapped himself to the wreckage with his braces. A woman had raised such a hue and cry at sunrise that she became exhausted and went under. At this point the play of the tropical sun on the horizon seemed to the remaining three of us to be the fires of hell. Their thirst was unspeakable. Adams, the radio operator, began to rant and mouth curses. Bob recalled how he remembered him:

> He spoke about all of us!—We would die of thirst and then drown like the others. I would drown, just like himself, no matter that he had cursed and I had prayed.... To be surrounded by water and to be dying of thirst—this was, indeed, a state of damnation!

Then he told me about all the things he had on his conscience. And finally, how he was about to be attacked by sharks, who were bound to be around there in their shoals. Mr. Bernardes had, in the meantime, expired. He was still held by his braces, and had simply died of thirst. I was already thinking that there is nothing for it… and then I thought that perhaps they are heading for us… yes, and Adams didn't feel like waiting any longer: "Before the sharks attack my living flesh," he said, and with that he reached for his knife….

Having arrived at this point in his flashback, Bob described in simple words the nature of his hope:

I was now alone but I kept on hoping. For something. For what, in fact? I didn't really know. Here I was in this total water wasteland. I was blind and could see nothing. But this was all the better, for I thought: Perhaps there will somehow be something that one does not see but which, nevertheless, is there. One has to hold on to some such belief. This gives one the strength to hang on. And this is essentially what matters.

At this dramatic stage of the story the reader can see the drift. Bob's report goes on to say that gradually the thirst affected his reason and so he began to drink the sea water. But, miraculously, it tasted fresh! His drinking the water was what saved him. The next day, a Norwegian freighter fished him out of the water and took him to port.

Bill, his young guide, was skeptical: "How could it have been that the water was fresh?"

Bob answered: "Ah yes, OK. I only found this out later. It was river water, even that far out in the ocean! You see, the Amazon, in the rainy season, disgorges an enormous amount of water into the Atlantic, with the result that the river water spreads for miles out into the ocean. That is how one finds such an expanse of sweet water in the ocean."

"And," retorted Bill, "if Adams had drunk from it he, also, would have survived?."

"Yes," replied Bob, "only he didn't do so. He had, beforehand, already lost all hope. And he was too afraid of the sharks. In fact, one never finds sharks where there is fresh water...."[1]

Tips for people with tinnitus and chronic illness

Suppose that you were one of the four survivors in the above story. Your burden, that is, the symptoms of ringing in your ears, is symbolized by the metaphor of thirst. Let us suppose it is hellish torture. But is it a situation devoid of hope? Do not imitate the woman passenger who used up her strength in crying (whether in protest, in fear, or in anger). Neither take the part of Mr. Bernardes, who "*was left hanging* in resignation." Above all, avoid the radio officer Adams model, who was, as it were, eaten up by nonexistent sharks. Rather, focus your attention on Bob and his ancient wisdom: Blessed are those who do not see, yet believe....

---

1   Helmich, W., & Nentwig, P. (1969). "Es gibt noch Wunder" from *Kurzgeschichten unserer Zeit*. Braunschweig: Westermann.

CHAPTER FIVE

Mind and Body Working Together

We have said that true hope is hoping against all reason, but, for all that, it is in no way unreasonable or meaningless. It brings about the paradox between the obviously irrational and the perfectly meaningful, as was the case of Bob being able to drink the sea water. Another relevant example is the last period of the life of the renowned lyric poet Theodor Storm. In the summer of 1887 his family doctor diagnosed him with an advanced state of stomach cancer. The doctor pulled no punches. Theodor Storm tried to deal bravely with this fate. Stoical composure, however, escaped him, and having to look on at his fast disappearing days weighed down his spirits. This melancholy influenced his poetry. The pain in the following lines is proof of this:

> With sounding step I walked the moor,
> Yet now that echo is weak, unsure.
> Fall has come, long past the spring,
> Was there then such joy and songs to sing?
> I would I were here today not in that past May—
> Life and love flow fast into the far away.

Storm went through unspeakable sufferings. Then hope took over and beguiled him to believe that another doctor, whom he had previously consulted, was the wiser one. That physician had diagnosed an expanded aorta, which was not malignant and would recede on its own.

Storm convinced himself that he had no cancer. He embraced life and began work on his greatest creation, the novel *Schimmelreiter* (*Dykemaster*). Storm achieved what no one thought possible—not even his family doctor—and finished his great work before he passed away on the 4th of July, 1888.

Does this mean that he had deceived himself? That's how it might appear, but hope knows better. Hope knew that if he had lost his confidence in life he would have deprived himself and the world of his exquisite spiritual study. No, he needed to put his faith in something that was way beyond the ken of the eyes of logic, and this faith bore fruit in his work of art.

As proof that all this operates beyond logic is that these examples cannot be generalized. One should not draw the conclusion that someone involved in a shipwreck can stave off imminent death by drinking sea water. In any particular case, what makes most sense and is most meaningful for a person "comes from above." Hope merely directs one towards the miracle.

The only conclusion of which we can be certain is that it is in the context of hope that the soul and body cooperate to best effect! Bob's body was the only one to hold out until the Norwegian freighter appeared, and this is not to be attributed only to his finding water to drink. The positive spiritual attitude of Bob's mind helped his body to hold out.

Strom's cancer-eaten body was enabled to mobilize its last reserves, but this was in no way due to the efforts of his family doctor. Storm's gushing inspiration enabled him to live on for a short time beyond his biological condition—nevertheless, it was exactly long enough. When the spirit is paramount, the body is slower to decline.

Ludwig van Beethoven, whose particular destiny allows us to include him in the series of our examples, wrote the following illuminating words:

> From where do I get my ideas? I cannot reliably say. They come unbidden, directly and indirectly; I can pick them up in my hands for free in nature, in the forest, when out walking, in the silence of the night, in the early morning, from the stimulation of moods that stir a poet to words but stir up tones in me, causing them to resound, murmur and build up to a storm, until at length the

notes stand there before me…. Yes, whatever is to touch the heart must come from above, otherwise they remain mere notes, a body without a spirit. What is a body without a spirit? Mud and clay. The spirit must raise itself from the earth towards the divine sparks that attract it. Somewhat like a field to which the farmer entrusts the precious seed, so that, by reaching out and up to the source from which it has come, it may blossom and bloom and bring forth fruit in plenty.[1]

One can therefore conclude that it was through some such hope-fired attitude that the deaf body of the composer was enabled to feed the inner hearing of his heart and spirit. By working together, *body with spirit* is capable of overcoming almost any handicap.

Tips for people with tinnitus and chronic illness

Similarly, you also can establish a bonding of your spirit with your body. This is achieved when you keep on hoping, if necessary, against all reason. But do not prescribe for your hope that towards which it must aim. One cannot force oneself to hope for a speedy recovery, the alleviation of hearing problems, or the like. Hope will instinctually believe in the miracles that are suitable to your situation. It assures you that such miracles happen, as long as you allow it freedom and do not interfere, either by rational arguments or by irrational fears and wishes.

---

1   van Beethoven, L. (1997). *Beethoven: ein Wegweiser für den Musikhörer in Zitaten und Zeugnissen.* Musicosophia-Verlag. pp. 35, 42.

CHAPTER SIX

How to Let Go of Fears

The full effectiveness of hope can be significantly impacted by irrational fears. A suspect whom fear causes to remain silent will make him- or herself even more suspect. A person suffering from compulsive hand-washing (ablutomania) who has an inordinate fear of infection may more easily pick up infection in overwashed hands than someone who has no such compulsion. A housewife expecting guests and in a panic about burning the roast will take it out too soon. The meat she will serve them will then be tough, thus in no way satisfying her guests. A child, who, out of sheer desire not to fail in his exams, attempts to make a cheat sheet and takes longer in doing so than would be needed in correctly mastering the original material. In this way the risk of failing is increased, and such a child thus becomes more unsure. Thus, the anxious person creates a world in which fear must reign—indeed, a world truly to be feared.

If one wishes, then, to escape these fears it is essential to let go of the pestering and (mostly) irrational anxieties. The two following examples invite our imitation.

First example:

One of my patients was firmly fixed on the idea that his wife would have a thrombosis. He had earlier read in some newspaper about the dangers of thrombosis, and when a small surgical intervention was envisaged for his wife his fear grew to an unbearable degree. On the way to the hospital he could already see his wife in the grave.

When he had admitted his fears to me, I asked him: "Tell me, what is your primary concern, is it for yourself or for your wife?" "Obviously, for my wife," was his immediate reply. "Therefore," I said, "the important thing just now is not what you expect, rather what is important is that your wife remains in good spirits and is not infected by your fears." My patient was able to see this. So I followed up: "Consequently it is your duty when you visit her in hospital to radiate a certain amount of optimism. But you will not be able to do this if you are quivering with inner fears. Therefore, leave aside your fears for the time being with the reflection: 'Even if my wife were to have ten thromboses, and indeed a heart attack as well, this will not prevent me from communicating to her that I am looking forward to our future together. For her sake I will keep my faith fixed on a positive outcome, come what may.'"

And this patient, with his eyes at once laughing and crying, by busying himself about radiating hope thus created hope within himself. Which hope was happily justified, for his wife soon recovered.

Second example:

A priest was terrified by the compulsive idea that, pushed on by the powers of darkness, he might masturbate in a church. Although he dealt with this as a fantasy produced by fear, which he would never really have carried out, he fled from his station and hid himself in shame in a hermitage. When he was brought to me I suggested the following plausibility: that God places more store in the solid trustworthiness of his earthly representatives than on a clean church building. He could prove his absolute trust in God by courageously entering the church no longer hindered by his fantasies. He would then, in fact, put up with the possibility that he might commit all sorts of indecent acts in the church, and then in simplicity trust that if such acts happen God, the "all-knowing," understood that he did all this from his disturbed state and not out of blasphemy.

The patient hesitated. I attempted to provoke him further with the question: "Or do you think that the God is not up to date in psychiatry?" He laughed. "You see," I said, "then go into your church with this laugh in the future, and if the fear sneaks back in meet it with the challenge—that He who knows everything can best distinguish between a harmless compulsive fear and a deliberate blasphemous act."

The priest went back to his post, and what haunted him melted away gradually out of his head, more or less unnoticed.

Tips for people with tinnitus and chronic illness

Overgrown, compulsive fears can be let go of if one courageously confronts the substance of these fears. This confrontation should be done with a healthy sprinkling of humor. The successful art of banishing fears ostensibly involves seemingly permitting the feared object to be magnified ("Even if my wife were to have ten thromboses…"; "Even if I were to do all imaginable immoralities…")—and thus de-emphasized—one is able to behave in a meaningful way. You can work out the most suitable way to adapt it to the symptoms of tinnitus or other chronic illnesses. For example: "Even if a whole orchestra were to be playing in my ear…" or "Even if I have to make friends with my illness…." In the face of such sovereign control, the fear will itself take fright, turn tail, and flee.

CHAPTER SEVEN

Cheerfulness as a Philosophy of Life

Let us examine a little more closely the "sprinkling of humor" just mentioned in the last chapter. This is a special class of seasoning which lends a neutralizing, sweet-smelling tang to the bitterest medicine. As distinct from a "rose-colored glasses" and "glowing colors" attitude, it makes for a human existence in a well-balanced cheerfulness, and this is a trait of the highest art of living

Even four centuries before Christ, the Greek philosopher Democritus wrote a treatise titled *On Cheerfulness*. By "cheerfulness," he meant an ascetic attitude of pleasantness and balance, as between too much or too little in all things. The phrase "ascetic attitude" indicated that we should so live as to accept tolerantly and without irritation the peculiarities, even the unpleasant ones, of our brothers and sisters. A clever bit of ancient wisdom! "Balance" referred to the idea that we should enjoy enjoyable things at least as intensively as we suffers from the unpleasant things. A further, equally clever bit of wisdom!

This immemorial notion of cheerfulness has an essentially deeper meaning than pure jollity. The cheerful person is one who has experienced the abysses of life and does not, through frantic straining, thereby turn away from life, but faces it head on with a laugh. Cheerfulness proves its worth in good times and bad: In good times, it is proof against silly and vaunting overconfidence; in bad times, against self-destroying withdrawal. It saves us from being a failure by trying to enforce good fortune from being broken by misfortune. It loosens what one might call our clinging attitude towards the earth and creates in us the necessary distance which puts us in a position to tackle confidently that which is changeable and to leave in peace that which is not changeable. Two examples speak to these ideas; a Russian anecdote and a Sufi story:[1]

First example:

As Khruschev was delivering his famous denunciation of Stalin, someone in the hall shouted: "Where were you then, Comrade Khruschev, when all these innocent people were being butchered?" Khruschev paused, looked around the hall and said: "Will whoever said that be so kind as to stand up!"

The tension in the hall began to rise. No one moved. Thereupon Khruschev said: "Now you have your answer, whoever you are. At that time, I was in exactly the same place you are now."

Second example:

A philosopher had an appointment for a discussion with Nasruddin, but he arrived at his house only to find that he had gone out. In a fury he took a chalk and wrote "Silly fool" on Nasruddin's door.

When Nasruddin arrived home and saw this message he hurried immediately to the philosopher's house. "I'd forgotten," he said, "that you were coming round, and I'm sorry that I was not at home. But of course I immediately remembered our appointment when I saw that you had left your name on my door."

In both of these stories, a person is the subject of attack. The accusation made against each one was not false, but rather harsh. Kruschev, while addressing his audience, was reproached with cowardice. Nasruddin was reproached with being a fool. At this point, then, the ball is in the court

1   Kornfield, J., & Feldman, C. (2003). *Geschichten, die der Seele gut tun*. Freiburg: Herder. pp. 103, 105-106.

of the accused. They can defend and justify themselves, which may arouse a new attack. Or they may counter aggressively, which might only serve to further damage them. Again, they can meekly acknowledge their guilt, which would serve to confirm the accusers in their harsh approach. They may decide to swallow their humiliation and take to their heels, the result of which might be stomach problems or headaches. Or they might....

Yes, they might also react with lightness, with a glorious mixture of acknowledgment of their guilt, dignity, mercy, and inner composure by nimbly and humorously batting back the ball. As the motto goes: "I'm weak, you're weak, let us mutually accept each other's weaknesses." Such a motto is a proof of strength.

Tips for people with tinnitus and chronic illness

And what about your humor? You also are being attacked. Besides unfriendly contemporaries, from whom you certainly will not be spared, you are attacked by symptoms of illness. Perhaps this is not totally undeserved—because of your lifestyle—but harsh. How about becoming a disciple of Democritus? Foregoing any unproductive responses, being ready to learn from faults, being happy about what is still intact and healthy, a gentle detachment towards what is not intact any more, and all this with a smile on your lips... surely, this is the art of living!

CHAPTER EIGHT

How Can Anything Become Good Again?

Whether patients are to blame for their own physical faults is never easy to tell. That there is no possibility that a person with sensitive hearing will ever get used to shrill and loud music is clear enough. That smoking too much, getting too little fresh air, eating too much, sleeping too little, watching too much television, not exercising... the fact that all of these burden the body has long been proclaimed. It was commonly held among the ancient Greeks, as noted in the last chapter, that too little or too much of anything was a health risk. However, not everyone's illnesses correspond to an individual's "sins"; indeed, many "sinners" live to a biblical age. An additional burden is imposed by the structures of our civilization, which are not tuned to biological fulfillment, but to materialistic demands.

If someone has to work under the simultaneous onslaught of diverse influences, that person cannot but experience some inner tension. Whoever practices a sedentary occupation has also to buy into its disadvantages. When someone has to do a long journey to and from work every day they are at the mercy of traffic troubles. It is possible, of course, to achieve an overall balance, but this demands much discipline, which is not always available.

When some deterioration in health manifests itself, those concerned begin to tear themselves apart in self-reproach: "If only I had...," "If only I were...." They turn to lamenting and focusing on the reason why, but it is too late. A patient of mine once said: "I have made a total mess, I just want to die." To this, I replied, "Should it not rather be that when you have done something wrong, it is *precisely* then that you need to go on living in order to undo this wrong?" She replied with a snort, "I cannot undo what I have done. Show me how I can make it good! Look at me: I'm a wreck. How can anything become good again?" She looked thick and puffy, her hair neglected, her clothes sloppy, unattractive, sick in mind and body. She had abused her powers over the last years, countless sleepless nights filled with black coffee and loud music, given restlessly to changing relationships, and investing no real care or interest in herself. The result of this was clearly visible in her trembling hands.

Characteristic of this situation is a struggle within the person. The person disregards, indeed hates, him- or herself. What this means is that there is one part of the person which disregards and hates, and another which is disregarded and hated. The first part will not stop disregarding and hating, as long as the second remains dull and stupid. This second part will not recover as long as the first ungenerously refuses to forgive. One of these two has to take the initiative in some action to break the vicious circle, that is to say, by offering "an earnest of love."

In a thoughtful mood I turned towards my patient. What part of her might best be able to take on this challenge? I did not know. Then I decided. I would read to her "The story of the white ribbons."[1]

> This story is about a young man on a train journey, who is
> clearly depressed by some problem. Finally, he confides in the
> fellow traveler sitting next to him that he has just been released
> from prison and is on his way home. His conviction had
> brought disgrace on his family. They never visited him in prison.
> Nevertheless, he hopes that they may have forgiven him. So he
> had proposed to them in a letter that they might give him some
> indication, as the train passed the family property, as to how they
> felt towards him. In the case that they had forgiven him they were
> to tie a white ribbon to the apple tree by the railway tracks. If they

---

1   From Fleischlin, P. J. (ed.). *In vaters garten*. [Publisher unavailable]

did not want him home they were not to do anything, thus he would remain in the train and travel on—somewhere.

As the train neared his home his excitement would not allow him to keep looking out the window. His neighbor promised to keep an eye out for the apple tree from his seat. Soon he laid his hand on the arm of the young prisoner. "There it is," he whispered, and tears immediately filled his eyes. The tree was covered from top to bottom in white ribbons! At that moment all the bitterness that had poisoned this young life vanished....

As I finished the story the eyes of my patient were close to tears. I asked her: "Tell me honestly now, into which role do you see yourself fitting: that of the young man, who hoped for forgiveness in spite of everything, and had proposed the same in his letter, or the role of the family, who overcame the old resentment and festooned the tree with the ribbons?."

"That of the family," she replied spontaneously.

"Fine," I said, "that is then your next assignment. You must stop blaming yourself, which you have been wrongly doing. Get yourself a small indoor tree and deck it out with a white ribbon, as you gently try to coax yourself by saying: 'Don't give up hope, many things will come right again. I like you and so I will be with you to help you. Together we will soon achieve this'."

This indeed did come about. The patient turned over a new leaf and attained an inner self-respect and a better outward appearance.

Tips for people with tinnitus and chronic illness

Perhaps there is also an empty corner in your house in which a small tree with white ribbons would look good. And might there be a corner in your soul where there is urgent need of a similar sign of forgiveness? Do not be too hard in judging yourself. None of us is born an angel, nor are we wisdom in the cradle. The particular circumstances that we have to bear are enough punishment for our sins. More good than we could ever allow ourselves to dream of can result from gracious gentleness with ourselves, with our lives, with our fellows and with our all-pervading fate.

CHAPTER NINE

Power and Responsibility

Here is another example of what one could call "dilemmas of conscience," gained from practical experience in psychotherapy. This is to show that self-acceptance and love of one's neighbor mutually stimulate one another, something which is fairly obvious already.

A foreign professor of geology came to seek my advice. He suffered from depression, which had recently worsened. Especially in the mornings, he just could not drag himself to undertake the simplest activities. For the evening lectures he felt fresher. Typically, morning "lows" suggested that a hereditary factor might be present. Indeed, the patient's mother had suffered from up-and-down mood swings since menopause, for which she had been treated with lithium. From this the suspicion was that his was an affective disturbance—an endogenous [biologically-caused] depression.

Because the patient had a scientific education and was an exceptionally intelligent person, I spoke openly to him about the suspected nature of his illness, and advised him to visit a psychiatrist with a view to getting some medication. I pointed out that his melancholy could be an emotional deception, as it occurs temporarily and without adequate cause on the grounds of neurochemical deficiency. Although he experiences his depressive moods as painful, he should at least hold on to the thought that from an objective point of view there is no external reason for his depression. His being and work remain meaningful, although temporarily he might subjectively think otherwise.

He looked at me earnestly and asked: "Are you sure that my work is meaningful?" His question made me sit up and pay attention. Was it telling me about insufficiency symptoms of an endogenous depression, or was it the cry for help of a man who suffered from a real moral dilemma? The particulars were clear and satisfactory, as I had ascertained from our conversation. He was respected in his college, he was an expert in his field, and as such made many trips worldwide. He was happily married with grown-up children who, in turn, had pursued respectable avocations. His doubts seemed to flow from some illness.

I replied: "Your work is meaningful in so far as you assess it *independently* from your depressive moods." He let his head hang and was silent. Intuitively I figured out: "Oh, so this man is wrestling with something other than his illness. He may indeed have an inherited melancholy but what really bugs him is an existential problem."

After a few minutes the patient replied out of the silence: "I teach my students how to find uranium deposits, through complicated analyses of rock samples."

My mind grasped things only slowly: Of course, surely geology students should be well informed about metal deposits, right? He divined my perplexity and explained to me: "Yes, certainly, that is part of the syllabus. And later when my students have finished their studies, they will be hired by industrial bosses to show them how to construct atomic reactors...."

Once more silence descended upon us, while his words reverberated within me. A scientist like this would hardly soothe himself with illusions. The main thing which presented itself to him as involving a terrifying risk is the disposal of atomic waste. What advice should I give him? That he give up his job? What a strange request! And what difference would it make? In such a situation would not another professor be installed in his place to teach the students exactly the same thing? The students… this was where I got stuck in my search for a solution. They were in pursuit of this knowledge, which they would pursue, in any case, in one university or another. One cannot withhold it from them.

The most important point is that, along with this knowledge, they should also acquire *knowledge about their responsibility*. This relevant connection is often overlooked. But who can bring this home to them convincingly? No one else except someone personally convinced about the responsibility of scientists—someone like the man who was sitting there before me!

"Professor," I said, "I would recommend that you lay your full predicament and your doubts plainly before your students. Explain how to find uranium, but pose them the question whether it is such a good thing to have discovered uranium. Not everything that is technically possible should be done, and this applies to geology also. Speak to them in your lectures about the question of *feasibility and responsibility*, and, before and above all else, you will gain in addition to the recognition of the scientific world, self-respect and the regard of your students.

"Yes, that is what I must do," the professor nodded in agreement. "Until now, I have been too inhibited. But yes, of course, that is how I must pursue my task."

Oddly enough, he was able to get through this whole thing without antidepressants, and when his period of depression had faded away, he became a fervent champion of environmental thinking. He was one of the first such from among the ranks of geological professors. It is easier to accept oneself if one loves mankind so much that in case of a conflict one is prepared to step out of line for them.

Tips for people with tinnitus and chronic illness

Moral dilemmas can push one into the arms of every slumbering symptom of illness. Your doubts can even make use of pathological symptoms in order to come from their hiding places to the clear light of day. They want to be heard, and for this purpose may even come up with a barrage in your ears!

Moral dilemmas long for your attention. So you hear inside yourself the plea "in God's name." What do you do, or leave undone, without the agreement of your conscience? Is there something there? Yes?

You should be aware that there is an alternative solution. When necessary, take the risk of stepping out of line. Stepping out is much healthier than letting your "hands hang limp."

CHAPTER TEN

Self-Conquest out of Love

The professor of geology primarily felt a certain inhibition in passing on his reservations to his auditorium. His healing came through self-conquest.

It is obviously true that self-conquest as an outer demonstration of strength is by itself not really virtue. People may conquer their shyness for utterly senseless reasons. Youthful hesitancy can be overcome by acting as a lookout for a robbery. Easy women can overcome themselves to share a bed with rich older men who flatter them. Young lads who hunger for sensation manage to overcome themselves so as to climb perpendicular walls with magnetic shoes. In a word, the *why* is decisive in assessing the motive for self-conquest. Very often shyness and timidity keeps us from follies and awkward situations.

Self-conquest will only appear in all its glory if it is achieved for the sake of someone or something else. When self-conquest is joined with love, the two combine to produce self-development of an exceptional quality. Self-conquest, when it focuses on *why* it is doing the act, strengthens and nourishes, "all-unintendedly," the self-conquering person. On this point I can offer a small but very rich example from my own teaching experience at Munich University.

One of my students was very shy. Most of the time she kept her head down; she blushed easily and never dared to take part in discussions in the lecture hall. In those days my custom was to leave the writing of lecture notes voluntary, and to take these into account for a student's final exam in case that student didn't answer enough questions to pass the exam.

One day, however, at the start of the lecture I forgot to ask who wanted to do the notes. Then the timid girl overcame her shyness to speak up and remind me of my omission. Immediately I replied by asking whether she might not be prepared to do it herself, and she, who had never before volunteered to do it, took it on. Months later at her finals she was one question short, but because of that protocol contribution she got through.

She certainly had helped *me*. But what came from this was a whole series of advantages to herself, namely, triumphing over her shyness, having the experience of doing the protocol, and finally the happiness of success in her exam. However, what was most beautiful in all this is that she had simply intended *to help me*. The purity of her motivation caused her decision to redound to her own advantage. Neither the crass egoist who is incapable of taking a step beyond self, nor the "I'd-gladly-be-a-martyr" who wants to "do everything right," could manage to attain such a result. While the egoist refuses help out of indifference, the "I'd-gladly-be-a-martyr" type will share indiscriminately and uncontrollably with everyone until he or she is exhausted. Often, the ideal lies in between. This ideal is that it be a sacrifice that is meaningful, performed out of love, the result of self-conquest, performed in the right place and at the right time, and for something or some person who needs it. Such a sacrifice does not burden the doer with exhaustion, but rewards that person with inner growth.

Recently in a newspaper cartoon, I saw a drawing of two kids before a computer. In his speech-bubble one kid was saying to the other: "When I go to school I don't know what will become of my mother, she can't even program the DVR!" A modern joke—yet, it was touching to note that the coming generation still has a heart for their parents, and that the robotic future will not deprive anyone of occasions of self-conquest. To be sure, the computer will not extinguish the imagination, the place where love has its roots. Otherwise, we poor human beings might undergo an inner shriveling rather than inner growth.

Tips for people with tinnitus and chronic illness

You will occasionally practice self-conquest, but do not offer yourself senselessly. Around you there are many people who are in need of help. Some of them you can certainly assist. Make an informed choice and proffer your service to them with a pure motive. And do not grumble aloud with: "And who ever helps me?" Do not do things with an eye to seeking thanks. Any return for yourself must flow freely, and not from your own preplanning. Your awareness that somebody else needs help already puts your own lot into perspective. Anything else that may then accrue to you by way of growth will be life's surprise for you!

CHAPTER ELEVEN

Uselessness—Apparent or Real?

To have an awareness of the need that is in the world around us is one of the best medicines for those who endure suffering. Normally, the swirling waters of self-pity for one's own suffering carry us to where we no longer notice any needs except our own. In opening up to the sufferings of a fellow human being, one also escapes the strong undertow and is carried out, so to speak, into less perilous waters.

The process of such a rebirth through tuning the attention was called *dereflection* by Viktor Frankl. Frankl recommended that, instead of *hyper-reflecting*—circling endlessly and secretly, pathologicially obsessing over either a momentary situation or a permanently incurable problem—one should direct one's attention to something specific outside oneself that can be healed; for example, to someone else's sorrows. Such a focus, on activities that have nothing to do with one's own pain, provides the troubled soul with some breathing space. Under the shelter of this dereflection, individuals are enabled to recover, to spread their wings, and to put a distance between themselves and their pain.

Many people intuitively make fruitful use of this method. Today, however, a modern trend goes against this—an immense and widespread resignation dominates. From this, is it possible to foreclose on the apparent uselessness of all constructive effort with the apocalyptic reasoning that *our world is ultimately beyond redemption.* The world is unstoppably overpopulated, environmentally polluted, ecologically out of balance, politically astray, and ruled by money, power, and corruption. Its continual destruction by human beings will exact its revenge on humanity.

In principle, these arguments are justified. Like every other species of animal, humanity will also die out. As with every other planet, the earth is cooling down. Sooner… or later… but does such a distinction really matter? It is at this point that the arguments begin to crumble.

The meaning of existence, especially a personal existence, cannot be based on its length, nor is it diminished by its transitoriness. This meaning has to have an anchor beyond any reference to time. Otherwise, the whole development of creation would resemble a frustrating Sisyphus operation after the model of that Greek tragic hero, who had to eternally roll a stone up the mountain, even though the stone kept rolling back down again. Many people in our current global upheaval identify themselves and our society with that ancient hero. This paralyzes them with regard to meaningful initiatives, and tempts them instead to close off any openings onto an apparently doomed world and to confine themselves to their own concerns.

This logic is a type of short circuit. Even the legend of Sisyphus is capable of positive interpretations. Perhaps the stone may be uninteresting, and is simply a means for keeping the hero strong and healthy. Perhaps the hero has some importance—he, the eternally young, because of his application to exercise, does not give up, carries out what is demanded, and goes along with the ups and downs of his fate. That which seems to be a punishment can often be an opportunity. As long as the stone keeps rolling, life is pulsating.

Let us add here another, more recent, story in answer to this challenge:

An old man was walking by the seashore as the sun went down. He saw a youngster in front of him picking up starfish and throwing them into the sea. When the old man caught up with the youth he asked him why he was doing this. The answer he got was that the starfish would die if left on the strand during the night. "But," said the old man, "there are miles of strand here and so thousands of starfish, what difference will it make for all your trouble?" The youth looked at the starfish in his hand and threw it far out into the saving waves. Then he suggested: "For this one, it makes a difference."[1]

Tips for people with tinnitus and chronic illness

Do you sometimes feel like Sisyphus? Do you throw starfish into the sea? Good for you, only more so, keep it up! Do not feign tiredness! Things that seem to be useless and futile may well work out best for you. Pay no attention to the whisperings of resignation, whose arguments can be tempting: "Whether you make an effort or not," it will whisper, "you are still a sick person, the noise in your ears persists. You still have many days filled with suffering in front of you. What difference will it make if you busy yourself today with another's troubles and forget your own?" Be happily strong like Sisyphus; look at your day—the starfish in your hand—and in the certainty of victory reply: "For this very day, it does make a difference."

---

1   [This story originated with Eiseley, L. C. (1969). *The unexpected universe.* Houghton Mifflin Harcourt. It has many variations; likely the closest version is Joel Barker's "The star thrower story," an archival copy of which can be found at https://web.archive.org/web/20070929155500/http://www.starthrower.com/star_thrower_story_script.htm –Ed.]

CHAPTER TWELVE

Sending Them Back to the Deep

We learned about dereflection in the last chapter, but we have not explored the full extent of its possibilities. Therefore, I will indicate another very important area of application. What we are dealing with is *post-traumatic stress disorder* (PTSD) and how to conquer it.

First, some information about PTSD. Those who have undergone a severe traumatic experience, such as a major shock from, for example, a war injury, traffic accident, an earthquake, or being taken as a hostage, are in a difficult and confused situation. On the one hand, they have graphically experienced how suddenly and unexpectedly everything can come tumbling down in ruins, those things that they have taken for granted each day. The fact that they have survived this ruination they often see as a pure gift. Nevertheless, it can be hard to establish a firm hold on the amazed gratitude and joy they feel at the gift of their survival. What very often stands in the way of such appreciation is what is called, in scientific language, *intrusion*. The basic meaning of this expression comes from a comparison with a volcanic eruption, where the burning lava explodes out of the bowels of the earth through the crust of the earth, and then congeals into layers in places where it does not belong.

Intrusion, transferred to psychology, carries a similar meaning. White hot snatches of memory in the form of flashing scenes, sounds, smells, which may or may not have been resolved, rise to the surface of consciousness even decades after the trauma, and because they are then out of place they interfere with current activities. They can influence the thoughts and stir up feelings for the persons concerned who, as a result, can easily feel out of control of themselves.

It must be noted that it is not true, as was suspected in earlier times, that people who are plagued by intrusions actually repress their traumas.

Studies have demonstrated that the vast majority of them were able to sensibly integrate their painful experiences into their lives, and that this majority were not in any way helped by reopening the old wounds through endless talk about them. On the contrary, the "magma" must be allowed to settle quietly inside the psyche—only that, unfortunately, it can congeal in the wrong places. Today we know why this happens. Every shock, because of an accompanying outrush of hormones into the blood, produces an immediate, corresponding, intense, superawareness (*hypervigilance*), by which every detail of the event is accurately recorded, as if forever happening. The whole context of the shocking event is instilled incomparably deeper than in other learning experiences, becoming virtually burned into the memory; such an engraving will not rest quietly in the storeroom of the memory. The drawer for the past in which things are stored is not, as it were, properly shut; the contents are all wedged together which is why these deep memories can slip back unbidden into awareness at some unsuitable occasion.

What remedial action can be taken? The answer lies in the use of dereflection through the setting up of a "refuge" in the realms of the creative imagination. People with PTSD are invited to name one of their most pleasant places of memory, which they are asked to describe in detail. For example, one individual described a hut in the wood where, as a girl guide, she had spent delightful hours of adventure. She described the moss-covered spruces and the thick ferns to the right and left of the door, the flickering candle on the rough wooden table inside the hut, and the sweet smell of roasting apples coming from the old stove. There, once, in a merry mood she had taken her recorder out of her rucksack and happily improvised tunes to her heart's delight.

She had now established as her refuge this idyllic memory of where she had been able to relax her body and rejoice her soul. Every day, she practiced this visit to her hut in the woods for a few minutes, even though it was only in her imagination. She could approach the hut at sunrise, in the snow, in a storm, in the gloom of autumn, and on any occasion open the door, go inside, light the candle and the stove, put an apple on the grill, and lie back cozily with her recorder.

"Here, I am secure," she would say to herself. "Here, nothing and nobody can weigh me down. Here I am in my homeland outside of time, beyond hardships, beyond death. It is wonderful to be here." When she had then drawn in a deep breath, and enjoyed her visualization for the length of a recorder tune longer, she would firmly return to reality.

Those who possess such a refuge can be offered escape from intrusions in this manner. They can rely on this immediate spiritual withdrawal as soon as the red-hot magma from bygone painful experiences comes sneaking back. This place of security will protect them from any trauma associations that may drop by. Quite simply, none of them are allowed in, so that they have to retreat back, defeated, into submersion in the deep. There they must be heroic and accept their eternal rest, back in the drawer of the past where they belong.

Tips for people with tinnitus and chronic illness

Are you also pursued sometimes by some shadow from the past? Are you buffeted with memory specters that come out of the blue and disturb your equilibrium? Do they browbeat you with pointless questions as to the why of your failures, nagging that surely a reckoning is bound to overtake you? Take an early flight to the land of imagination! Transport yourself into this most beautiful realm easily prepared by your imagination. It will give you a safety that is out of this world. Inside there we will glimpse pictures that may well be more real than those our minds can grasp. In this place, you are totally safe from the unacceptable memory specters, and the *why* question fades, unasked.

CHAPTER THIRTEEN

Sending Them Ahead to the Waiting Room

According to a law of psychological health, the objects to be dealt with by our minds and emotions should be attended to "in their turn," then and only then. There are times for looking back: Things of the past can be mourned or celebrated, or perhaps both. There are times to look ahead: Things of the future can be looked forward to or feared, or perhaps both. But above all, there are times to be in the here and now of the present, while you are in the midst of life itself.

It is only in the present, when we are most alert and intensive that we are able to actively take part in the construction of our own and others' lives. The past is enclosed in history and unchangeable, the future is uncertain and enveloped in a fog of a thousand possibilities. The present alone can still be changed because it hasn't yet quite happened; we are fleetingly, as it were, granted the privilege of choosing one of the thousand possibilities and adding this to the truth about ourselves.

What a pity it is, then, if we lose out in this serious consideration of the present, as happens with the problem of intrusion which was just described. By dwelling on pains in the past, we can miss out on present opportunities for joy. In dreaming about past joys, we may squander the opportunity for renewal and revitalization. Likewise, it can be a pity if forethoughts dominate, as indeed sometimes happens: People feel they must be ever planning, or grieving, or brooding about what terrible things may happen; they are coming to grips with the gloomiest possibilities. Or they float in Utopia, living with storybook princes and princesses who end up in thin air. All this is not healthy. There is no doubt but that it is good to be orderly! Issues of the past must be sorted out, assessed, and (like file folders) be archived. They are not the focus of attention in the present. Possibilities of the future have to be critically illuminated and then allowed to nestle in trust. This is also not the time for that. The present should be freely accessible, unclogged, and fresh—nobody should be tripped up by things left lying about!

Whoever keeps the past and the future clear and sorted out is in the best position to be devoted fruitfully to that which *is to be dealt with here and now*. A gynecologist once approached me, looking for help. He had a somewhat compulsive disposition: fearful, pedantic, perfectionistic. His medical practice was giving him financial headaches, though it functioned like clockwork.... "Until now..." was all he could say. He feared that, with the new health reform and a new accounting system, he would go bankrupt. He was also picking up hints that his own strength was weakening. What if he should drop from exhaustion? If he had to temporarily close his practice, he would lose some faithful patients. He did not know how long he could sustain the stress. His nights were spent tossing restlessly in bed as he searched for ways to safeguard his income, and then there was his family....

I broke into his lamentations: "Doctor, I would like to pose a question to you. Let's suppose you are busy at a consultation with a gynecological patient. Suddenly, two impatient women come storming from the waiting room into your consulting room looking for immediate attention. What would you do?"

The doctor wrinkled his brow: "I would send them both back post haste to the waiting room," he replied curtly. "I could not allow them to interfere with my work."

"Exactly," I laughed, "you make it clear to the women: 'Out, it's not yet your turn!' Isn't that so?" Slowly what I was trying to say began to dawn on the doctor, and a smile spread over his face. "Now," I continued, "say exactly the same thing to your fear-inspired anticipations when they come sneaking in. You must shout at them: 'Off with you, into the waiting room until later, it's not your turn! When my practice is really in trouble *then* you may make your way in here, and *then* I will reflect about solutions, but, in the meantime, do not interfere with my work!'"

The gynecologist was delighted. "That is an excellent idea, I must do just that," he beamed. "From now on, all that has nothing to do with the present will be sent back, or rather sent on ahead, to the waiting room which is the future. What a liberation!" From then on, he was once more able to have a normal night's sleep and to concentrate during the day on each case as it presented itself. His practice began to flourish as it had done before.

Tips for people with tinnitus and chronic illness

Are you also sometimes bothered by fears about the future? Do these buffet you with terrible specters that suggest to you how hopeless everything is, and what dreadful things are about to happen? Your symptoms of tinnitus will become more piercing, simply unbearable; your bodily infirmities will get worse and worse, they will render you totally helpless; do such thoughts keep spinning about in your head? Please, usher them out politely into the waiting room of the future! These apparitions can have a seat and bore themselves by leafing through the magazines. It is only when the appointment time for one of them comes up that it will put its case before you. Until that time, you will be left in peace—and by then you will have built up enough strength to deal with them!

CHAPTER FOURTEEN

Time Brings Many Surprises

The old saying "Time will tell" is not devoid of wisdom. The time laid out before us, which is this "time that brings," contains even more surprises. In this regard, the following is an interesting exercise: Let us write down what was of utmost importance to us ten years ago, what intrigues we were plotting nine years back, what had us on our toes eight years ago, what seemed to us especially worthy of our efforts seven years ago, and so on, up to the present.

How do these momentous things look to us today? Several will have fallen into the background or will have been settled. One or two will have become absurd or childish from today's point of view. What one absolutely had to have then is, to some extent, now only lumber. What one once could only dare to speculate about in one's wildest dreams is now commonplace. Perspectives shift with time.

If we took this into account, we would get less worked up about many things. We would remain calm like the philosopher in the following story from Novalis:

The Philosopher

"Teach Homer to my canary," said the tyrant to the Philosopher, "so that he can recite him by heart, or else you must leave the country. If you take on the job and do not succeed, you will have to die."

"I will teach him," said the Philosopher, "but I must have 10 years to do this."

"Why were you so stupid," his friends asked him afterwards, "as to take on something impossible?"

He replied, with a chuckle, "in 10 years' time either myself, or the tyrant, or the bird will be dead."[1]

Eugen Roth was attempting to express something similar, (but the other way round), in his own charming fashion, when he took issue with the extreme health freaks. These want to prevent the evil of disease and yet are powerless once their last hour approaches:

Pointless striving

A man once longed with longing to stay alive
Saying death with him would have to strive,
His first thought was to keep strict eye
On self, and so survive his call to die,
Secondly, that he might stop the rot
By serious scientific plot.

For him the science to enlist
Was horoscope of astrologist,
That never planet on his side
Should dare to wander or collide.
With Saturn numbered in his cast
He added the help of his good gymnast,
That turning torso and bending knee
Might issue in certainty and bring him glee.

By food uncooked his vitamins save,
Nor wine nor smoke make him a slave,

---

1   Werle, von J. (Ed.). (1998). *Deutsche Fabeln aus tausend Jahren*. Munich: Goldmann. p. 218.

His hormones so would wildly fly
His years and face to re-beautify.
His life and sap were soon united
To science and to cooking dieted.

A man like this must gain his worth—
To live one hundred years on earth;

But—fate by none is obligated
Nor will she retreat her claim unsated.[1]

What is the common note in these two very different texts? "Ten years on today's problems are just empty words," is Novalis's message. Eugene Roth teaches us that "for all our foresight, there is no way we can get a peep at what is in store for us." For all our efforts to arrange our affairs, important things may turn out differently than expected when the time comes. And, in any case, death always decides on a closing time earlier than we have planned.

But it is not just negative surprises that are in store for us. In 10 years' time, it may be that tinnitus will be completely curable. Illnesses like cancer, AIDS, multiple sclerosis, and so on, may then have been deprived of their sting. Medical advances are exploding—but whether for the common good remains to be seen. Does fate, which cannot be opposed, find itself here and there thwarted by this progress? In 10 more years, the world of mores and culture we know will be different, and ourselves with it. What distresses us today may then be unimportant. As well, there may be many new joys in our lives that are now totally foreign to us. In the end, cute little robots will take on our unpleasant tasks, and their artificial intelligence may thus add some variety to our loneliness. Who knows, who knows?

So let us remain alive with curiosity, open-minded, and ready for surprises, never overestimating our state-of-the-art achievements. The river of time brings many things into perspective.

---

1   Roth, E. (2002). *Eugen Roth für Zeitgenossen*. Munich: Carl Hanswer. p.21.

Tips for people with tinnitus and chronic illness

When the tyrannical symptoms of tinnitus make impossible demands on you, react with philosophical composure and set about gaining yourself some time. In a few years' time a chip may be invented that, when fitted in the ear, will cancel out the noise. So there is firm hope that the tyrant will be dead before you are!

Nevertheless, you must never forget your finiteness. We cannot expect immortality from the wonders of medicine! Death is what is in store for all the living. But above all, do not reduce your life span by making desperate efforts to lengthen it. Rather, adorn your life with the shining light of love, and rejoice in the life span which has been granted you.

CHAPTER FIFTEEN

The "Aha!" Experience
of Seeing Things From the Other Side

The two-sidedness of things, that is their ability to fluctuate between opposites, is rooted in their relativity. This can cause us trouble, because as human beings we need fixed standpoints in relation to which we can locate ourselves and ideas that serve as guideposts by which we can figure out our way. Complexities and ambiguities make us feel decidedly uncomfortable.

This two-sidedness can also produce conflict. Contrary standpoints anchor people in conflicting positions. Someone who does not share our view can appear as a threat. The one whose views we don't share appears to us to be on the wrong track. It demands the consummate art of real tolerance not to fall into primitive thinking and label others as "enemies" when confronted with this ability to fluctuate.

Here is a striking example of the two sides of one and the same situation, taken from a brilliant film about big game animals in the wilds of central Africa. The film first illustrates the dilemma of a majestic family of lions during a long period of draught. One sees the noble beasts wandering about for miles in search of prey. But the hunt is in vain, because all the suitable prey have already died from thirst. The lions are gradually using up their energy, getting thinner and thinner, until finally, reduced to skin and bone and with their manes all matted with sand they lie down wearily under a bush. The sympathy of the viewers is totally with them. Then the hoped for reprieve draws near: a herd of elephants approaching through the steppe. The lions would never have dared to attack them, but luckily for them one weakly, worn-out, mother elephant trotted along behind the herd.

What happened next is a testimony to the intelligence of the hunting beast. The lions jump to their feet, put their heads together as if in quick consultation, and split into two groups. One group hops in between the mother and the herd, at once to distract the mother and at the same time to isolate her further from the herd. This is what promptly happens. Then the other group presses forward out of ambush and make their deadly attack.

Bravo! The film audience breathes a sigh of relief, now the lions have enough food and especially blood to drink and so survive.

But this sigh of relief was of short duration. The scene shifts back to the beginning and focuses on the elephants. Now we are looking at the herd tromping through the dried-up desert, with nothing green in sight. The elephants are famished. But the most distressed is an in-calf mother, dragging herself along, weighed down with the added burden of her calf. Soon the time comes for her to give birth, but the baby is too weak to live.

The next shots would draw tears from any audience. The mother elephant tries to make her baby stand up and shake itself into life, as she pushes it gently to and fro and massages it with her trunk. She doesn't want to "believe" that it will never move. All the while she is losing contact with the herd, and because of her lack of strength can't keep up or close the gap when she finally drags herself away from her dead baby. All the sympathy of the film audience is now with her as she hurries to her fate in the shape of the brutal lions.

It is an eye-opening experience to place ourselves in a position from which we can see both sides, in this case the view from the lions' side, and then that of the elephants. Not only does it shatter our preconceived biases, but it widens our basic range of understanding. Indeed, even the bright sides of our human existence are not without shadows, and conversely our darkest sides are ever subject to flooding by flashes of light. This is surely to gain a huge insight! One has only to occasionally change sides to have access to such invaluable "Aha!" experiences.

> **Tips for people with tinnitus and chronic illness**
>
> Do you rate your chronic sufferings as a huge misfortune? You are right! The beasts in the film were also correct in feeling their sufferings. Nature does not despise the right of creatures to complain, and further she enfolds it with the gold of the complementary side. The lions released the elephant from her misery; the elephant saved the lions with her blood. And what is the complementary gold intertwined with your tinnitus or other chronic illness? Out of your resilience, shift your standpoint, and then you will find it. You may well then be able to assert: "Yes, looked at in this way my misfortune was fortunate… it saved me from… it got rid of my…."

CHAPTER SIXTEEN

The House With the Golden Windows

On the subject of being "wrapped in the gold of the complementary side," here is another symbolic story:

There was a man who lived in a tiny house. He could have been content with his life, but every morning he went on about finding a better life. As he looked out of his window, his eyes were drawn to a house across the valley. This house had golden windows that sparkled like diamonds. How he would love to live in such a house! The idea so fascinated him that one day he made his way over to the house with the golden windows. He took with him all the money he had saved up, so that perhaps he would be able to buy the house. The path over was especially difficult. How disappointed he was, then, to find at his arrival that the house did not have golden windows but ordinary panes of glass.

Exhausted and tired, he sat down in the evening sun and looked back in the direction of his own house. And how amazed he was to realize, in the brilliant evening sun, that now his own house had golden windows![1]

It is hard to miss the message of the story; the only question is how one translates it into real-life examples. Does each person really have to agonize through all the steps described above? Must envy, discontent, and lack of

---

1   From Fleischlin, P. J. (ed.). *In vaters garten*. [Publisher unavailable]

self-respect gnaw at individuals until they make a breakthrough and succeed in dispelling their longings? Must people be ruled by the absurd idea that they can acquire contentment for money? Must human beings puff and pant along a difficult path in order to find out at some stage that they are chasing after a mirage? Must one first be matured through means of bitter disappointment at the deceptions of life before turning back (reversal, remorse, repentance), and, from the distance attained in the meantime, become aware of what divine spark has been granted to the little bit of existence that oneself is?

In the psychotherapeutic dialogue according to Frankl, one finds a characteristic question to pose to the individual to cut through the difficulties involved in this awareness process. It runs like this, with some possible variations: "What would you do if you did *not* have these cares or problems, that is to say, what would you do other than what you are now doing? How would your life differ from what it actually is now?" Or, in the terms of the above story, "If you were living in the house on the other side of the valley and the windows were golden, what difference would this make?"

It is always exciting to be able to hear the answers. It is only those who have a clear and precise answer to this question that need help to bear with their sorrows, or need support in solving their problems. More often, individuals are taken by surprise, embarrassed as to how they may reply to this question: "*how might it be if...* if one were not handicapped, if one were loved and respected, if one were more fit and stronger, if one's troubles were to cease? Would that be heaven on earth?" They are not convinced of this. Of course it would be better to be healthy than sick, rich rather than poor, and so on, but... what then? One's ideal life cannot be best described in terms of the absence of difficulties.

Therefore the question "*how might it be if...?*" requires us to re-examine all of our basic tenets, and that may lead us to the realization that it is best to be at home within oneself, provided the windows are not curtained against the sun.

Tips for people with tinnitus and chronic illness

Do not waste your energy in peeping over other people's fences;
do not allow yourself to be dazzled! The houses at the other side
of the valley of pain also have only plain, ordinary windows. What
you should consider instead is what you would make of your life
if you had no noise in your ears or no burden of chronic illness:
What would you set about doing? Who would you embrace? What
musical enjoyments would you indulge in? What tasks would you
achieve? And now be honest with yourself: Do your symptoms
really stop you from doing these things? Is it not true that most
of these would be somehow possible if only you had a conviction
about how much gold shimmered on your own house? If, simply...
you were content?

CHAPTER SEVENTEEN

A Question to Think About

I will never forget the day, at a conference in Kansas City, (USA) when I was asked to demonstrate a therapeutic dialogue. Full of good spirits, I readied myself to do so. When the patient was finally brought into the room I found that she had only a few weeks to live, because she was suffering from throat cancer which was progressively blocking her breathing. In fact, for this very reason, she had to have an oxygen cylinder always at hand. My optimism soon vanished and gave way to a feeling of helplessness. What possible comfort could I give to this woman?

After mutual greetings, we sat together in silence for a few moments. During this time, while I was in a state of bewilderment, this credo came back to me, one that has so blessedly accompanied me throughout the decades of my professional work: Every human life is permeated with meaning, literally to its last breath! Like a wave out of an agitated sea it welled up from out of my reflections and feelings and gave me strength. I looked into the face of this doomed woman and began our conversation.

We started with a consideration of the precious things in her life and established that no power could steal these from her. She described in detail a rich variety of common and uncommon experiences of her life, centered on her highest value, her extended family. Children and grandchildren were all brought up on her farm, all closely bound to the ancestral land. Sons-in-law and daughters-in-law were received into the family, and the different generations all got along with each other. Two more farms had been acquired, the herd modernized, and a great-grandchild was on the way. As I listened to the words of this woman, I could understand how she experienced saying farewell as difficult.

At this point, something suggested itself to my lips: "Did you say that, until now, none of your children or grandchildren was ever seriously ill? And that no major accident had ever happened in your family?"

She looked at me pensively. "Yes," she replied, "we are, thank God, an unusually healthy and strong family. Apart from the usual, like a broken leg, an appendix, and so on, my husband, brothers and sisters, and my children have been spared until now. I am the first one to have such an illness, I alone...."

For a time, out of grief she struggled for air, but this short period was sufficient for me to carefully consider my therapeutic approach.

"So you are the only one to have such an illness," I said, linking in with her words. "On this point may I pose you a question? Assuming it to be simply impossible that such a big family as yours should remain fully free of illness over the years, and supposing it were too much to demand of fate that no mortal illness should touch even one member of such a big family, suppose then that you could choose which one of the family it had to be who would fall ill in this way, *which one would you choose*? A brother, a daughter, a son-in-law, a grandchild...?"

"Heaven forbid!" shouted the woman, with some of her former energy vibrating in her voice. She drew her upper body up to its full height. "No," she explained firmly, and as she spoke she seemed in a strange way to gain in strength, "if one of us were to get ill, if one of us has to be the first to go, then *I would like it to be me.*"

"So then, if the choice had been yours...."

She would not allow me to finish speaking. She affirmed with total certainty: "If the choice had been mine I would have chosen what fate has chosen for us." Thereupon, the whole group assisting at the conference broke into spontaneous applause. It was marvelous. Everyone present witnessed how a human being under mortal threat could say "yes" to fate.

Theoretically, then, there is an alternative to every distress, which may please us even less than the distress in which we find ourselves. From this perspective, the possibilities of suffering are open-ended. The American farmer was not enthusiastic about her throat cancer. But if she were to remain healthy while one of her daughters died, this would have distressed her much more. If ever we have to call our fate in question and are faced with such an alternative, our protest will tend to soften towards acquiescence.

Tips for people with tinnitus and chronic illness

From early in human culture, there is a myth that says it is possible to deal with distress and pain through an act of self-sacrifice: "O God, accept my suffering and my renunciation, and in return protect those who are dear to me."

In these or similar words, countless numbers of faithful ones have pleaded down the centuries. The patient mentioned above had also indirectly done the same by unhesitatingly placing herself as a shield in front of her family.

And what about you? Listen to your deep inner voice: Do you perhaps find some resonance of this myth within you? Do you see yourself folding your illness into a sheaf for sacrifice, to the accompaniment of your tinnitus cacophony? On behalf of someone else who means a lot to you?

CHAPTER EIGHTEEN

Keeping One's Eyes on the Lighthouse of Meaning

We have come to the end of our tour through the aids available in Frankl's psychology, although there remain countless other comforting gems of wisdom, ancient and new, to be found there. As explained in the introduction, there should hang at every crossroads a signpost with the inscription: "Take this road only in time of stillness." In this way we will not pass things by.

Without stillness, our "antennae" remain inactive and deaf to what is right for our humanity; not even the voices of angels could reach us.

On the other hand, in the concentration that is supported by stillness, our antennae can pick up, figuratively speaking, the very echoes of the Big Bang, the morning chorus of creation.

It is for this reason that the meaning of our lives, which is a meaning independent of our present miseries, can be deciphered only in moments of pause, of letting go, and in being still. Whoever decides not to put this into practice will never escape the din of this world. Such an individual will soon experience the tragic comedy of the following Sufi anecdote:

> Mullah Nasruddin was on all fours under a street lamp outside his house when a friend came by. "What are you up to there, Mullah?" asked the friend.
>
> "I have lost my key and I am looking for it."

At this, his friend also went on all fours, and they both spent a long time poking around in the dirt, under the lamp, looking for the key. When there was no finding it, the friend turned to Nasruddin and asked: "Where exactly did you lose it?

Nasruddin answered: "I lost it in the house, but there is more light here under the lamp."[1]

Indeed, meaning can be found not only in the light, for very often one has to seek it in the dark. However, it must be precisely in the place where we have lost it. One has to find one's way back—perhaps even on our hands and knees—to where one went astray.

A patient of mine was a man who held a very high position. He slaved at his job until he was half dead, leaving both his body and spirit burned out. He soon needed to have a clinical examination. Asked why he had not slowed down sooner, he said he thought it was because he had decided to force himself to complete the major project he had taken on at work. However, he was not able to keep it up through willpower. In the meantime, the all-important deadline had come and gone. He was shaking from the frantic pressure, and cold sweat covered his brow.

At this, I asked him for a totally honest report as to how he experienced that project, and it became clear that he rejected it internally, because he saw it as, in his words, industrial hubris. He could see no sense to it, but now that it had been taken on, he decided to carry it through to the deadline. I now invited him to admit that he *didn't* want to do even this. This was the reason why all his willpower was eroded, because basically, he did not see why he should invest energy in something he regarded as unsuitable. At the same time, I forecast to him that, after his rehabilitation, so long as he dedicated himself to projects that fitted in with his personal convictions, he would not have any further physical or mental breakdown.

---

1   Kornfield, J., & Feldman, C. (2003). *Geschichten, die der Seele gut tun.* Freiburg: Herder. p. 36.

This man, therefore, had to look for the key to his healing in the place where he had lost it, his workplace. Accidentally I learned that indeed that was where he found it. Some years later, I met up with him in a department store. He looked radiant and was in great form. He had changed his job, he told me, and now worked, on contract, at political research, which interested and satisfied him. He often did overtime in the evenings but it did not tire him, and he felt no resulting ill effects on his competence, as he had in the past. Gently and almost a little shamefacedly he added: "Who knows? I might still be sitting at my old job if I had not had my nervous breakdown." From this experience he had found this "meaning within darkness."

In truth, meaning does not always turn up as the companion of our lively enthusiastic days. Rather, it is often as a lighthouse in a dark and stormy night, when the little ship of our life is rudderless, and threatened with upending. It appears like a messenger of the gods to keep us on our course. It is the call which invites us in through the door of life.

When do we become aware of this shining glow, this attracting call? When we are still and quiet. And when are we really still? Not when things are silent, but when the noise of the world does not bother us, nor tinnitus, nor illness, nor throbbing anxieties within, nor murmuring squabbles without.

Whoever has inner quiet is sound and whole.

A final tip—for everyone[1]

If it be your wish
To enter the door to life,
You must set out, and discover the road,
Which figures on no map,
Nor is described in any book.
Your feet will stumble over many stones,
The sun will beat down
And thirst will burn you,
Your legs will begin to drag.
The burden of the years
Will weigh you down.
But at some point
You will begin to love this road.
Because you will recognize it as your way.
You will stumble and fall,
But you will have the strength to get up again.
You will take roundabout ways and go astray,
But you are coming ever closer to your goal.
Everything depends on
Your risking the first step.
For the first step
Takes you through the door.

Wolfgang Poeplau

---

1   Poeplau, W. (1983). *Geh durch das Tor zum Leben*. Freiburg: Herder.

Part B

Reflections on a Psychotherapy
With Dignity

CHAPTER 19

The Meaning of Life and Goals in Life for People With Chronic Illness

It is one of the fundamental logotherapeutic principles: Life has an unconditional meaning, which cannot be lost under any circumstances. Viktor E. Frankl not only maintained this, he lived it. He witnessed that one can say "Yes to life" under the worst conditions; for example, the conditions of a death camp during the Second World War.

For our generation, death camps are fortunately not the problem. However, in every society, even in wealthy ones such as those in the northern hemisphere, death is a part of life, not only as a natural finishing point of a person's history, but also as a lifelong threat for us all and especially for those of us who are incurably ill. Of course, medicine has made tremendous strides; on the other hand, modern man's lifestyle has become much more stressful and insane, and the pollution of our environment in its widest sense has reached such a high degree that the incidence of handicaps due to accidents and chronic illnesses due to a weakened immune system has risen within the population despite medical progress. Thus modern knowledge and technical instruments are able to increase our life expectancy, but not necessarily the quality of life in proportion to that.

A lot of people still suffer from imprisonment in a sort of "death camp," one not built by political enemies, but instead by fate, the fate of a damaged body, which does not allow free planning for a personal future. How can we support such people in defying feelings of hopelessness, resignation, self-pity, and doubts about the meaning of their existence? How can we help them to understand, that their presence in the world is not in vain, is not a mistake of creation or—even worse—a torture, a punishment from above, but is as important and basically wanted as every human life on earth?

From puberty, the point in time when the personal self takes control of the individual, we make blueprints and plans for our lives. These plans are changed again and again in a dynamic process; they are permeated with ideals, reconciled with realities, enriched with hopes, and rebuilt on buried illusions.

Despite these ups and downs, a constant line can usually be seen, a leitmotif that everything else follows. In the individual psychology of Alfred Adler, one speaks of the finality of human efforts; in the transactional analysis of Eric Berne, of the respective personal script.

Our plans for the future reveal as much about us as does our past. Although there often is a great discrepancy between what we intend to do and what we have done, this discrepancy reveals characteristic things about us. Accordingly, in order to understand who their clients are at present, psychologists should draw their conclusions not only from what these individuals have experienced and how they developed, but also from their plans.

Of course, the past already has become certainty. Nothing about it can be altered or changed. The future, on the other hand, is uncertain. Corrections are still possible and goals can be changed. Nothing may turn out as we believe it will. If one were to compare our past life with the pages of a diary in which no erasures or rewrites are permitted, then our future plans could be compared with the outline of an essay for which an unknown number of empty sheets are available with the condition that the pen not be held by our hand alone.

These considerations have relevance to Frankl's concept of meaning:

> Man resembles the flier who is "piloted" into the airport through nocturnal mists to make a blind landing.... The marked course alone leads the pilot to his goal. Similarly, every man in all situations in life always has marked out before him a single and unique course by which he can attain to the realization of his most personal potentialities.[1]

The meaningful path

In this quote, there is no mention of "predestination," because the pilot does not need to submit to following the invisible glide path that guides him safely to the runway. We are free to steer, free to veer off, even to switch off the engines and go straight down (as is every suicide victim). However, if we want to arrive where we ought to arrive, where conscience and responsibility direct us, where it is best for all concerned, then we must freely commit to this designated path, for this is the most meaningful path.

Likewise, there is a most meaningful path for every person, with signposts to unique tasks that we—and only we—can and ought to fulfill. All human beings are awaited by something in particular which can and ought to be theirs; there is something intended for each of us in this world, a world that *we never would have entered were we not welcome here.*

Just as a safe spot on earth awaits every aircraft, wherever it takes off, and a dear friend or a personal task awaits each passenger at the destination, every person on earth has a great love or a great work waiting for them that is theirs alone to choose, to activate, and thereby to transcend their own temporal existence.

We set our own life *goals*. How we do this depends on internal factors, such as mental state or character structure, but the *meaning* of life enters our lives from without, is assigned, designated, and addressed to us; it is a guiding ray that leads us to the highest realization of a unique, irrevocable personal existence.

---

1   Frankl, V. (1986). *The doctor and the soul.* pp. 55-56.

This view of meaning offers a comforting perspective. Consider this: Is a glide path conceivable that would guide a jumbo jet to a tiny airport with a runway far too short? Is this not unimaginable? It would be senseless to guide an aircraft to the wrong airport. In the same way, there can be no task intended for us for which we do not have the necessary time, strength, and talent at our disposal.

If a meaning in life truly awaits each person, then everything that we require for its fulfillment must lie in our cradle from the beginning. And if an individual meaning of life awaits each person, then something different must lie ready in each cradle, a different supply of abilities, opportunities, health, and time. A plane which is near its destination needs very little fuel; a plane whose destination lies high in the mountains needs deicing equipment. All of this must be taken into account beforehand; otherwise, the plane is not cleared for take off. We, too, cannot be cleared for take off into life with a designated path that we cannot travel unless we postulate a cynical, sadistic image of God, which I will not assume here.

In psychotherapeutic practice, patients who have adopted this view can succeed in becoming calm and composed with respect to their plans. A teacher who was in counseling with me drove to a principals' conference saying to herself "If it is I who am supposed to represent the interests of our school, then, with proper preparation, the necessary energy and skill will come to me. And if the necessary energy and skill fail to come to me, then this task is not my task, but is intended for someone else; I will gladly withdraw from it. After all, other people want to be good for something too." Six months earlier, the same teacher had been terrified of participating in the conference and of suffering some lapse for all to see.

A further example is an individual with a chronic illness who had long hesitated to begin a course in social work. The question, "As sick as I am, will it be worth it to take this course?" had always held her back. After counseling, she decided to begin immediately despite this and not to waste any more thoughts on whether she would live long enough to work as a social worker.

She had understood: If this was the meaning of life awaiting her, then hours and days would be there for this activity as a social worker. It could not be otherwise. If the necessary hours and days were not there in the end, this would simply mean that no activity in social work awaited her, and that the path laid out for her would find meaning and fulfillment in the training itself, full of interest and joy.

In order to rise to this inner calm and composure it is necessary, however, to take to heart two aspects of the point of view described:

1) Even if I can be sure that I possess the power to travel the path designated for me, I cannot succumb to the error of thinking that the path can be traveled without effort on my part. The meaning of life can long remain hidden even when we look for it and does not land in our laps; it must not only be sought, but also conquered. Only when I contribute my share of effort, commitment, practice, and (of course) take care of my health and fight any illness, only then will that which is intended for me be realized. Without my efforts, it remains pure potential, a good path that could have been traveled.

2) That which is not present in me as potential is not mine; this bitter truth must be accepted. How bitter it is depends on my attitude. Some people protest against blocked paths, but who knows how steep these paths would be? Drivers complain about closed mountain passes in winter, even though this is done for their protection! Similarly, a particular task could be too difficult for us and is therefore not intended. Therefore, let us see it as a relief that our days and strength are limited. Otherwise, there would be so much more in the world for us to concern ourselves with, to worry about, to take on.

Life goals

Life goals are set and chosen by the individual; they bear the unique stamp of their designer. They are created, despite periodic adjustments, with relatively high consistency. The pattern according to which we forge our life plans changes much less often than the plans themselves. As noted earlier, all life goals and life plans are uncertain, as part of the future, they are the outlines of diary pages still unwritten, the contents of which are not in our hands alone.

Now let us try to build a bridge between a) the meaning of life as the guiding ray of providence that invisibly but perceptibly pervades our lives and b) personal life goals that are visible in acts of will and in wishes, but of which we can lose sight. The bridge consists of the awareness that the nearer our life goals approach the life meaning which is present from the beginning, the more certainly they will be achieved. This is expressed in the following formula: *The more meaningful a life plan, the more probable is its completion.*

What argument comprises the main supports of this bridge? Simply this: Since all internal capabilities and external opportunities for realizing our plans are "placed in our cradle" in order to fulfill that which awaits us, we are optimally equipped to aim at goals within the realm of that which awaits us, and ill-equipped to pursue aims that lie beyond these goals.

Of course, we can set goals that do not correspond to the unique meaning of our unique existence, but when we reach for that which is not meant for us, we must be prepared to fail. The pilot who leaves the glide path assigned to his route to fly in darkness and fog to a distant airport of his choice increases the uncertainty of a safe landing.

The healthy and the sick

All of our considerations to this point are equally true for the healthy and the sick. The difference between them is not great, for, to put it bluntly, both are condemned to die. Both have limitations of strength and time. Perhaps the only difference is that the healthy can always become sick, but the sick cannot always become healthy, so that a step towards death is possible under all circumstances, but a step in the direction of life is possible only under certain conditions. Just as the past is more "certain" than the future, death is more "certain" than life—a fact far more apparent to the sick than to the healthy.

Whether their goals must therefore be of a different nature must be investigated. Since the healthy have no guarantee of an unlimited life, they cannot build their life plans on greater security than the sick. The certainty with which a plan can be put into action is based not on a presently stable constitution, which can be reversed at any time, but on the congruency of our plans with the unique plan which is intended for us. For this reason we must ask: *Is it possible that something different awaits chronically and terminally ill people?* Is it possible that something essentially different is intended for and assigned to them, a meaning of life of a special quality? If so, then their self-set and highly personal goals might be different from those of the healthy.

This question is not easy to answer in theory. Here are two examples from practice.

In the first example, I had a client who had a bad marriage. He came to me to talk, or, more precisely, to complain. For two hours, he grumbled about his wife. Since I always like to hear the other side, we arranged an appointment for his wife. Before this could take place, however, the couple had a car accident in which the woman was thrown from the car and seriously injured. She sustained brain damage and remained paralyzed on one side of her body after spending months in hospital.

Her husband, who worked, placed her in a good nursing home and maintained regular contact with her. He visited her every other day, caressed her, read to her, fed her, washed her, and took her outside in her wheelchair. He often brooded, feeling a mixture of regret and guilt about his earlier married life. Then he came to me because he couldn't break loose from this brooding. "Why did my wife and I get along so poorly?" he asked me. "Why did we bicker constantly about trivial things?"

How can one reply to this? It's the old story of the flowers one should give during life, because their fragrance is wasted on the grave. But in this case, life was still present, even if it was encumbered by disabilities, and the man was giving flowers, both literally and figuratively, by caring for his wife. This deserved emphasis. Thus I spoke of the "flowers of the present."

"I'd like you to consider one thing," I began. "If your marriage had been happy, then what you are now doing for your sick wife would have been a matter of course. It would have been the logical consequence of a happy relationship. However, what you are doing is something extraordinary, an amazing achievement. Now, you could easily take revenge for the many small disagreements with your wife. You could make this human being, now helpless, atone for any nagging and quarrels with which she may have made life hard for you. But you do not do this. You fulfill your duty as a husband, independently of what once passed between you. This demonstrates inner greatness. And you could never have put to the test this inner greatness which you possess if things had been different. You would not have known of its existence. You would never have discovered what tremendous ethical potential was dormant within you. Only in this constellation: bad marriage–accident–permanent helplessness–dependency of your wife on you—and *loving care by you for your wife*, only in this constellation has something in you been revealed of which you can be proud."

The man had listened, deeply moved. When I stopped speaking, he came closer to me and whispered his reply as if it were a confession. "To be honest," he whispered, "it is her inner greatness that makes that possible. She bears her fate calmly and patiently. Every time I walk through the door, she smiles radiantly. She never takes out a bad mood on me. I have no idea how she manages it, but she shames me so much with her attitude that I am changing from day to day, following her example. The ethical potential of which you speak leaps from her to me like a spark; I can feel it."

The second example concerns a 12-year-old boy who had suffered from leukemia since he was nine. His father was a doctor and I met him at a medical convention, where we talked. I asked him if it was difficult as a doctor to have a chronically ill child, for whom he could do little more than relieve his symptoms while watching the illness progressively worsen.

The doctor thought about this. "You know," he said finally, "sometimes it seems to me that we have gained more through our son than we have lost through his illness." This statement fascinated me and I asked him to expand on these thoughts. He then told me that his wife had suffered from symptoms of depression for years. Since their son's 10th birthday, however, she had been healthy. What had happened? She had asked the boy what he wanted for his birthday and he had replied: "A happy mommy!" Wringing her hands, she had sobbed: "How can I be happy when you are ill?" to which the boy replied: "But mommy, if I can live with my leukemia, then so can you. Just accept my illness as you accept me." Obviously the mother thought this over and had fulfilled her son's birthday wish.

But this was not all. The doctor continued: The boy's siblings and the children in the neighborhood had also benefited. They had become more sensible and mature through contact with his son. His son had, for example, given a nearly new football that he could no longer use to a child who had been ostracized by the other children because he came from a disadvantaged background. Since then, the unpopular child had risen in the group ranking by several steps and was tolerated and even liked. They had learned to help the weak instead of laughing at them. "You have mentioned your wife and the children who, as healthy people, have practically been taught by your sick son," I said, spinning the thread further. "What about you? Have you received any insights from your son?" "I?" the doctor asked, at a loss for words. "I have received the most. I have rediscovered prayer."

Opportunities for individuals with chronic illness

These two examples are not exceptions. They are part of a bigger picture. What is reflected here? What can we conclude? Individuals who have chronic illnesses obviously have a greater chance to exercise an "instructively converting influence" on those in their environment. This sounds remarkable, but it corresponds to the facts. The word of those concerned is genuine. The statements of the afflicted are believable; their suffering grants them a position of trust to which no healthy person can lay claim.

If I stood up and announced that one can reconcile oneself to leukemia, I would appear ridiculous. A 12-year-old son was able to proclaim this message with ease. His mother, siblings, the children in the neighborhood, and his father accepted it from him without resistance. If I stood up and announced that life with brain damage, one-sided paralysis, and confinement to a nursing home in a wheelchair was still worth living, I would be attacked by critics and skeptics. Yet, the wife of my patient demonstrated this clearly every day.

Thus there are perceptions, not to say "wisdoms," which can be conveyed only by certain groups of people simply because they would not be believed from anyone else. Thus this favored group of people is called upon to use this opportunity that has been placed in their hands for the good of others. It could be a meaning of life which is assigned to them and meant especially for them, for if they do not use this chance, no one else can use it for them.

Frankl, who is not only a neurologist and psychiatrist but also a survivor of four concentration camps, has spoken out all his life against the theory of the collective guilt of the German people. He gave a now-famous speech, the gist of which was:

A Jew must go and confirm that there were both kinds of people under the Nazi regime, decent people and unprincipled people, and that it would be unjust to condemn them all, lock, stock, and barrel. Non-Jewish Germans do not have the authorization, so to speak, to proclaim this truth, since they would be accused of trying to smooth over Nazi atrocities. No, a Jew who has suffered cruelly under the Aryan henchmen must go and confirm this. Then the next generation will understand that there are only two "races" of human beings on earth, namely the decent and the unprincipled, and these are present in all peoples and cultures, societies and nations.

I often hear similar statements from specialists who work with drug and addiction therapy. Who has the right to demand from those who are addicted to alcohol or heroin that they do without their drugs and bravely endure the withdrawal symptoms? Those who have never been addicted have no conception of the journey through hell they are proposing.

A former addict who has been saved and has escaped this very hell is fully entitled to say that the torment of withdrawal is worthwhile in spite of everything, because outside, beyond the condemnation to eternal dependency, waits the freedom of a life with dignity. Those who have been rescued can impart the certainty that rescue is possible.

Those who have an illness as an inspiration

The initial question was: Could it be that something completely different awaits those who are sick, especially those with chronic or terminal conditions—a meaning of life of a special quality? Practice grants us insights into an impressive perspective. People with chronic illnesses, and only these individuals, can bear witness to the mental and spiritual capabilities possible under the most difficult conditions. They and their families, who are also in a difficult situation, can testify that the internal acceptance of the inevitable is possible and that peace with the world and with the noölogical dimension is attainable, even if the illness remains incomprehensible.

When individuals with chronic illness formulate and demonstrate their "Yes to life," their positive model can inspire thousands of healthy people who may despair of life and, when they bear their fate courageously, through their example they may motivate thousands of fearful people who are afraid of life. Those with chronic illness and their families could be our best teachers, showing those of us who are healthy the true values in life. These values are not performance and success, competence at work, or expensive self-realization at any price, but rather much simpler achievements such as coping with everyday life without grumbling, gratitude for small joys without being embittered by pain, consideration for each other without losing our patience, and much more.

In what direction would a society of people, bursting with health and strength, drift if it were not for those who have illness, who are aged, who have disabilities who caution us to reflect on the true values of life? In what monstrous overestimation of itself would humankind land if we did not have guardians of the knowledge of our limitations and defenselessness?

The fact that such "miracles" are usually preceded by a long process of crises and depressions does not detract from the shape which finally emerges, of which Viktor E. Frankl noted: "Life does not take shape until it has endured the hammer blows of fate under the white heat of suffering." The suffering does not detract from the shape that finally emerges from the hammer blows. On the contrary, it imparts a "halo" to these guardians of a humanity that tends to overestimate itself. In any case, they have long done penance for any errors or slip-ups under the "hammer-blows of fate."

Our patients give us a plain hint. Those with chronic illness are called upon and asked to testify that life is unconditionally worth living and affirming, for *nobody can testify this as they can*. They are called upon and asked to do this in the interest of everyone, the healthy and the sick, the happy and the desperate; between health and sickness, contentment and need, there are flimsy walls whose collapse no one can predict. That is the special meaning of life for those with chronic illness. All life goals that they may set for themselves will always be within reach insofar as they answer this call. Whether these goals are related to professional or family life, education, activity, friendship, experience—for every one of these goals, the required time and strength will be available to them. Thus they will express, through their attitude and radiance, the truth that the courageous approach has value in itself. For, in the end, what counts in human life is not success and profit, but rather the true values, which are simple but nevertheless real. One does not need a long life to testify to this.

Reflections on the agave

On my last lecture tour in Israel, I saw once again those Mediterranean agaves which bloom only once in their life cycle. They inspire me every time to a brief reflection.

For a long time, the agave sprouts and increases by sending out shoots. However, at the height of its growth period, it produces a straight stalk, as stiff as a tree trunk, on the tip of which the blossoms unfold as in a flame. The rising shoots fall to the ground, exhausted. All the sap now flows to the blossoms which are to develop into fruit. The agave becomes drier, dustier, tougher, but it holds up its trunk-like stalk with iron roots long enough for the fruit to ripen and for the seeds to be scattered. Not until the wind has opened the last fruit capsules and carried off their contents does the empty stalk collapse. With it, the agave dies.

How our lives resemble these agaves! Our lives are by no means concerned with escaping collapse and death, but rather with the *upholding* before our collapse and death *that one essential thing*, pumping all strength into its blooming and ripening, and finally with opening the fruit of our life so that the wind which blows through time and space can carry it beyond our narrow sphere to where it can continue working when we have passed on. Thus it is the goal neither of human beings nor of the agave to live a long life. It is our common goal not to live for nothing.

In this similarity there is, however, one difference. For the fruit of one agave may be replaced by the fruit of another. But the fruit of one human life remains unique and irreplaceable. That which has been withheld from the wind that blows through time and space is lacking in the world and makes it a breath poorer in value. Let us therefore not be concerned with the withering in and around us and with the falling calendar leaves of our days. Let us look at that which stands straight in our lives, held high by the roots of our existence. It is *this one straight, flaming thing*, spreading itself out, which makes all collapse and death small in the face of greatness and makes collapse and death acceptable at the end of our way.

A foreign body forces itself
into an oyster
and creates pain.
Gritty sand rubs and
makes soft parts sore.
The oyster suffers.

The oyster tries to expel
the foreign body
but it engulfs
the grain of sand firmly,
thus making it impossible
to get rid of its pain.

Then the animal creates,
as part of its
instinctive wisdom
the power to change
its suffering
into a triumph—

From discomfort and need,
from the secretion of tears
arises
after a long process
of inner growth:
the pearl.

Elisabeth Lukas

CHAPTER 20

The "Birthmarks" of Paradoxical Intention

O ccasionally, the question is raised about whether the psychotherapeutic technique of paradoxical intention has anything to
do with the concepts of logotherapy. In my years of practicing
logotherapy I have never doubted that paradoxical intention is a true child
of logotherapy, even though it is frequently adopted, under various names,
by other schools of psychotherapy. Its logotherapeutic origin, however, can
easily be identified.

Paradoxical intention has characteristic marks—one might call them
birthmarks—that reveal its origin and account for its success. Behaviorists
use certain paradoxes that do not possess these birthmarks; their interventions produce similar, but not identical, effects in reducing symptoms. It
is my hope to clarify the connections between paradoxical intention and
the logotherapeutic view of human nature, and thus to eliminate all doubts
about the conceptual origins of this successful method.

Change of attitude

One of the birthmarks of paradoxical intention is *the phenomenon of
change*. Logotherapy might be called a great "quick-change artist" because
it succeeds again and again to transpose the meaningless into a meaningful

situation or to elicit a value from apparently meaningless events. In accomplishing these changes, logotherapists know the real connections. Their "tricks," if they are used, are based on a knowledge of human nature; otherwise, they would not work.

Paradoxical intention, however, does not produce "trick changes" in surface behavior which can be easily manipulated, as is often believed. In contrast to other techniques in the arena of psychotherapy, paradoxical intention brings about a change of inner attitudes, not temporarily but rather as a lasting new attitude toward oneself and one's feelings.

Paradoxical intention brings forth a calmness in the individual, a return to a basic trust that has been lost, a fundamental confidence that things will fall into place even if we do not always understand how. Paradoxical intention brings about a humility that has almost religious undertones—the realization of our own shortcomings, which are embedded in a universal order of meaning. A person who can say, "All right, if I have not locked my door, then let it be open, wide open, so a whole procession of thieves can walk in and rob me blind," is made to feel the relativity of all possessions and material values and is gently reminded that we are mere specks of dust in the works of the world and of time, and that our presumed treasures are insignificant within an infinite universe. An individual who smilingly imagines presenting a boss with a sizeable puddle of sweat or bombarding a superior with a broadside of stuttering babble is someone who has realized that there is a higher authority than the boss, and that the boss is merely another human being.

Individuals with symptoms of phobias and obsessive–compulsiveness suffer from a distorted perspective that makes close-up details appear frighteningly large and important while more remote goals, being apparently out of reach, seem insignificant and not worth striving for. Such individuals are like children watching a street from a high tower, mistaking the crows circling nearby for giant monsters, and the trucks on the street below for toys. The morning toilette becomes a complex ceremony; the bus trip to work, a frightening journey; the desk at work (which requires constant orderliness) a tremendous time-stealer; a sharp word from a coworker, a major crisis… that's the small world of the person suffering from these symptoms. In such cases, there's no room for the large outside world, which presents a continuous challenge to the human spirit.

Paradoxical intention puts details in their proper places. During the morning toilette, those millions of bacteria "sitting all over the skin, must not be splashed with water so they won't get angry as a wet hen." The bus trip provides time for a little fainting spell to make up for the lost morning sleep. A hurricane is invited to sweep over the desk to send pencils dancing. And the coworkers with all their remarks can go to hell.

The profound testimony of these exaggerations is the ridiculousness of wasting precious minutes of our lives on such trifles instead of saving our emotional reactions for important things that remain unattended. Without a change of our inner attitudes, without a shift of our attention from the small to the big, paradoxical intention cannot be accomplished. Therefore, the emphasis of this method is on the word *intention* and not on the technique of the paradox which is used, in many variations.

An experienced marriage counselor once told me that he has kept many couples together by advising them to separate. "People love contradictions," he said. "The grass is always greener on the other side. If individuals are forced to stay, they want to leave. Once they leave, they want to go back." There was some truth in what my colleague said, yet he applied the paradox only as a trick. Once, I assumed such a paradoxical position with a wife who spent hours complaining about her husband. I agreed that her husband indeed must be the "most cruel, incompetent, unlovable, and evil man in God's creation." She immediately stopped her complaints and began to talk about some of his good points. The crucial difference was that she *knew* my words were not meant seriously, and she was gently admonished by my exaggerations to correct her inner attitude toward her partner, to not exaggerate his minor faults. If I had advised separation, she might have found the idea appealing. A trick may or may not work, but a change of attitudes that will help a person get a perspective is always a gain.

Logotherapy was by far the first and, for a long time, the only psychotherapy that paid attention to attitudes. The emphasis was so strong that it assured attitudinal values a permanent place in psychotherapy. Addressing attitudes is a focal point in a therapy plan that leads individuals with psychological symptoms back to normalcy. The attitudinal change from a hyperfocus on unimportant details (which characterizes those with symptoms of phobia and obsessive compulsiveness) to a remarkable disregard for the unimportant, thereby opening the door to the meaningful things in life, is a common logotherapeutic concern which could have originated in no other concept of human nature.

The self–self dialogue

Another birthmark of paradoxical intention is *the dialogue with oneself.* The call to "know yourself" has been heard in psychotherapy from its inception, and it was commonly thought that all problems would be solved by self-knowledge. The call has become more subdued. Self-knowledge turned out to be a slippery concept; the more that contradictory evidence was found in the depth exploration of the psyche, the more the original enthusiasm vanished.

Meanwhile, practitioners of logotherapy quietly found a better approach to the self. Attention was focused on influencing rather than understanding the self. This approach is more effective because it is active. Its results are more tangible than those produced by interpretations and fantasies to which we fall victim when we explore the unconscious and the subconscious in a search for "hidden forces." A meaningful self-to-self dialogue is only possible if we conceive of a dimension of the spirit (where the self is in control) with a dimension of the psyche (where it is controlled by those hidden forces).

This view of the human being is a prerequisite for the discovery of the human capacity for self-distancing and its use as a tool in therapy. Only when logotherapy offered this view did the idea emerge that the self could be used in its own training.

The idea of "influencing the self" has been enthusiastically received and many books offer advice on how to achieve it, mostly without crediting its logotherapeutic origins. One of the best examples came from the founder of logotherapy in the form of paradoxical intention and its self-self dialogue between the spirit and the psyche. "Good morning, grouch," one individual will say to himself when he wakes up in the morning, depressed and in low spirits. "Go ahead and spoil my day. We'll see if you'll succeed! But put a little effort behind it, will you? It's no fun fighting a pushover." "Now finally I have a good reason to get mad," another person will say after having dropped a cup of coffee. "I always get mad with no good reason, now I can enjoy my anger because it's justified!" Such short dialogues with the self immediately chase away the negative mood which, paradoxically, was intended.

I have had clients who freed themselves from their fear through an inner dialogue with the fear itself rather than with the feared consequences, which is the rule. But some phobias are so vague that their consequences are hidden in a fog of nebulous threats. In such cases, individuals can be encouraged to ask themselves: "Where in the world did I leave my fear today? It would be awful if I had lost it somewhere and couldn't find it any more. It's been my steady companion for so long, I'd miss it terribly." These vague, abstract fears are more prevalent today, in an age of daily reports about nuclear and ecological disasters, than they were in the past when those afflicted with symptoms were afraid to blush at the wrong moment or to have sexual failures.

Therapeutically, it is easier to get patients to wish to "become as red as a tomato" than to wish for poisoned oceans. All the more important is a paradoxically intended self-to-self dialogue which can counter even vague fears.

Without the capacity for self-distancing, there is no reasonable basis for a dialogue with one's self; who is to talk to whom if there is no perceptible distance between the noëtic and the psychological self of one and the same person?

The concept of self-distancing legitimizes paradoxical intention as a true child of logotherapy because this method constitutes 90 per cent of a therapeutic dialogue with the self. This legitimacy is not invalidated by the many practices used by other schools which do not admit the paternity for methods strikingly similar to paradoxical intention.

Humor

A third birthmark that identifies paradoxical intention as a child of logotherapy is *humor*, the ridiculing of symptoms that is like a psychological volcanic eruption. Only rare patients have a sufficient sense of humor to see through the tragic aspects of their situation and appreciate the comical side of the paradoxical formulations. But once they see the ridiculous behind the tragic, they begin to laugh and keep laughing, not only about the nonsensical formulations that they are to repeat but, above all, about the fact that, after all those long torturous years of vainly fighting against their fears and compulsions, they are able to break the neurotic vicious cycle with a simple trick. (It is, however, neither simple nor a trick). They laugh about themselves, their fears and compulsions, their paradoxical intentions; they laugh themselves healthy.

"I cannot travel by train," declared an obese client. "I always have to think that I'll open the car door by mistake and fall out." "Why by mistake?" I asked, paradoxically intending. "Why don't you make up your mind to open it occasionally and fall out a little? There is no better way of reducing than somersaulting along the embankment—you probably don't get enough exercise—falling off the train is your great chance because then you can jump back in again and you'll see how those extra pounds will tumble off you!"

The person laughed, and at our next session was still laughing: "I took a train and every time I looked at the door I had to think of your crazy prescription to reduce, and the fear went away. Such nonsense...." The client broke off and began to laugh again. This person had no more difficulties traveling by train.

In what conception of human nature does humor have a proper place? From what theory of human nature can it be derived? I know only one: the concept of human nature, expounded by logotherapy, that recognizes a specifically human dimension oriented not toward pleasure and pain but toward sense (and nonsense). Sense and nonsense are the anchoring points on which humor is fastened like a balancing wire. This client could not have balanced across that wire of humor without knowing of the deeper sense in my "nonsensical" words, that falling out of the train was not possible without the desire to fall out.

When we laugh about a joke, we laugh not about a nonsensical string of words but about the kernel of sense behind the nonsense in which we perceive a meaning; we "understand" the joke.

Paradoxical intention must be humorous or it becomes a dangerous autosuggestion. Think of what would have happened if the client, instead of paradoxically intending, would have made the autosuggestion to fall off the train! By the use of humor, paradoxical intention becomes part of the meaning dimension of the human spirit, and thus draws closest to the source of logotherapy. Humor is not only a birthmark of logotherapy, it is its distinctive feature. Those who can laugh about their symptoms have already begun to overcome them. They are carried off, from their sickness and misery, on the wings of the spirit, which remains unaffected by the torments of the psyche.

I run.
Fear—
it comes closer.
Fear—
I flee.
Fear—
it catches up with me.
Fear—
I scream.

Fear—
it is here.

I stop running.
Fear—
I turn toward it.
Fear—
I approach it.
Fear—
I laugh at it.

Fear—
it is gone.

Elisabeth Lukas

CHAPTER 21

A Validation of Logotherapy

L ogotherapy is difficult to validate because it concerns itself with the dimension of the human spirit (the noëtic dimension) in which individuals are free to take a stand toward—and even against—all measurable factors and limitations of their biology and psychology.

The biological dimension—the concern of medical therapy—is the area of the electrochemical and physical life processes, which are visible, testable, and repeatable. Research is more difficult in the psychological dimension, the concern of psychotherapy. The substance of the psychological dimension is invisible and must be measured or estimated by projections and manifestations. Observations, emotions, and the intensity of drives are highly subjective. Even so, a substantial amount of regularity and interdependency has been reported, especially by behavior therapists.

But in the noëtic dimension the area of freedom is so immense that it has been doubted whether scientific research can be carried out here at all. The individual's capacity to accept, ignore, or oppose the limitations of body and psyche seem to make empirical research questionable.

And yet, despite a person's freedom and individuality, there exists a regularity in the human dimension. Frankl called it "the will to meaning." My own term for it is the *meaning postulate*. The prerequisite of human health and inner satisfaction is that human beings perceive their actions as meaningful, that they see a goal to reach for or a value to actualize—in short, they see a meaning in their existence and thus do not vegetate aimlessly up to their death.

The meaning postulate is the only firm condition to be found in the highly diversified area of the human spirit. In order to explain and justify logotherapy, a connection between the meaning postulate and health must be demonstrated.

The Logotest

The *Logotest* (Lukas, 1972, p.233)[1] was developed from the answers of 1,000 randomly selected persons on the streets of Vienna. They were asked whether they considered their lives to be meaningful and, if so, in what areas of their lives they found meaning.

Of those questioned, 51.0% stated that their lives had meaning, and 11.9% replied in the negative, 20.9% were inconclusive (9.2% walked on without answering, and 11.7% declared that they were still searching), and 15.7% indicated a negative answer without expressively saying so (3.0% ridiculed the question, and 12.7% rejected it). It was assumed that at least half of these two groups, by their cynical or negative attitudes, could be added to those who had found no meaning in life. When this was done, a total of 19.8% had either stated outright or indicated that they felt their lives had no meaning [see Table 1]. This table parallels clinical research that concluded the noëtic origin of all neuroses at around 20%.

The results of the groupings were used as the basis for the Logotest. The test consists of statements to which meaning-oriented persons would answer positively, and those in existential frustration negatively (Lukas, 1972, p. 62). After running measures of validation and statistical significance, a test was available to indicate the degree of a person's positive life content or, conversely, the danger of a noögenic neurosis.

---

1   Lukas, E. (1972). "Zur Validierung der Logotherapie" In *Der Wille zum Sinn*. Bern-Stuttgart Wein: Verlag Hans Huber.

	Percent		Computation in Percent	
Cannot see positive meanings	11.9	all	11.9	
Ridicule question of meaning	3.0	half	1.5	11.8 negative
Reject question of meaning	12.7	half	6.4	
Refuse to answer	9.2	all	9.2	
				20.9 inconclusive
Still searching	11.7	all	11.7	
See positive meanings	51.0	all	51.0	51.0 positive

The replies of the 51% who answered positively were grouped by meaning areas:
> Personal well-being (happiness)
> Self-actualization
> Family, children
> Career
> Friendships
> Interests, hobbies
> Experiences (nature)
> Service in a cause
> Overcoming distress (hunger, sickness)

Table 1: Logotest interviews with 1,000 people in Vienna

In an extensive scientific investigation lasting almost two years, the Logotest was applied to 340 persons: 285 persons randomly selected and 55 patients from the psychiatric clinic at the University of Vienna. All of these individuals were adminstered other psychological measures, using strict criteria to check the reliability of the results.

The three most important interrelationships are illustrated in Figures 1, 2, and 3. The connecting lines indicate a least significant difference of 1%, which means a probability of 99% [that the findings did not occur by chance –Ed.]. The three illustrations confirm the assumption of logotherapy that the well-being and stability of a person is related to how meaningful life is to him or her.

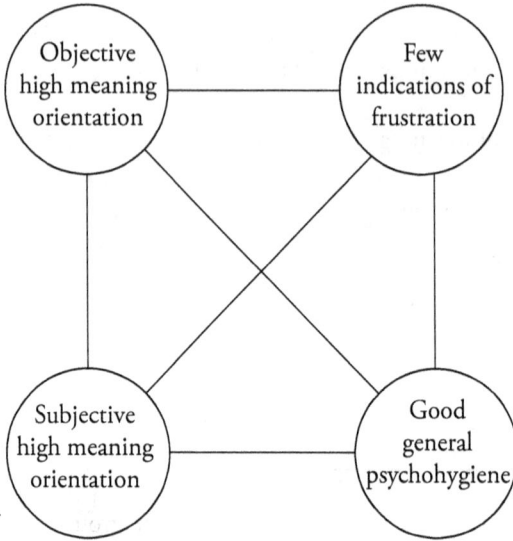

Figure 1

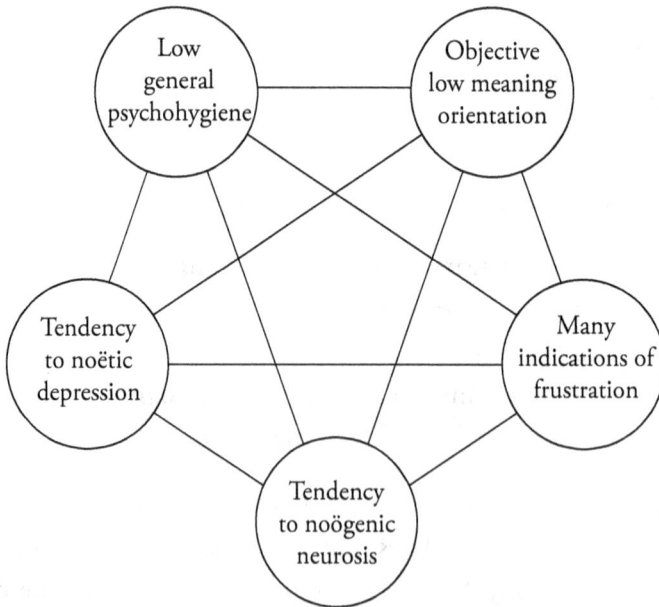

Figure 2

The interrelationships shown in these figures are not coincidental concurrences but interconnected factors: If any one factor is left out, there is a high probability that the interrelationships between the other factors will no longer be present. The illustrations show a regularity within the human dimension of the spirit, the only regularity that is demonstrable in the face of individual freedom—the basis of logotherapy: the meaning postulate.

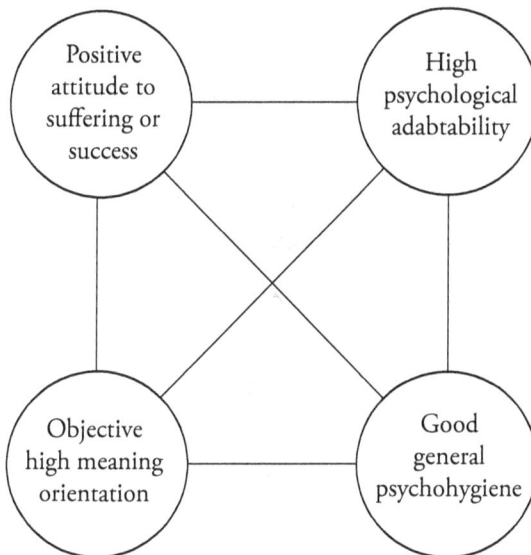

Figure 3

Premises[1]

From my own and other empirical investigations emerge the theoretical structure of logotherapy:

Axiom: The human being possesses a noëtic dimension.

From this axiom, a number of premises follow. I will discuss six.

---

1   [These premises, and the methods of logotherapy, are presented in far more detail in the fourth book of this series: Lukas, E. (1984/2020). *Meaningful living: Introduction to logotherapy theory and practice.* Charlottesville: Purpose Research.

Premise 1: *The human being has three dimensions*

(This assumes that the dimensions of soma and psyche—biological and psychological—are granted).

Premise 2. *In each of the three dimensions, the dependency on given circumstances is different.*

    A. Within soma, the biological dimension, the dependency on given circumstances is almost total and hardly manipulable.

    B. Within psyche, the psychological dimension, the dependency on given circumstances is flexible and highly manipulable.

    C. Within the noëtic dimension there exists the possibility of a free decision of attitudes to given circumstances.

Premise 3: *The three dimensions form an inseparable unit.*

Premise 4: *No dimension must be disregarded in psychotherapy.*

From this premise follows the obligation of the psychotherapist to include consideration of the question of meaning. But "also" does not mean "exclusively." The fourth premise simply says that the therapist must treat patients in their totality, and that therapy must include all dimensions, at least marginally. The minister must not be limited to religious wisdom when a member of his congregation comes with family problems. The surgeon must not confine attention to the amputation of a leg when a patient suffers from bone cancer. And the psychologist must not be restricted to the interpretation of test results when a client questions the meaning of life. All members of the helping professions have an obligation to respond to a genuine call for aid, if not on a professional level then on the human level. If they feel incompetent in a certain area, they must refer the person to others who can provide adequate help.

Premise 5: *In each of the three dimensions, the feedback mechanism works differently.*

    A. Within the biological dimension, feedback mechanisms bring about automatic processes (such as in the autonomic nervous system) that help the body adapt to the changed situation.

    B. Within the psychological dimension, feedback mechanisms bring about reinforcement processes and lead to changes of behavior.

C. Within the noëtic dimension, feedback mechanisms bring about changes in self-understanding and lead to a new interpretation of the self.

Premise 6: For each of the three dimensions, the principle of homeostasis has a different validity.
A. Within the biological dimension, the homeostasis principle is always valid.
B. Within the psychological dimension, the homeostasis principle is valid most of the time.
C. Within the noëtic dimension, the homeostasis principle is not valid.

Nearly all theories about human nature see homeostasis, the absence of tension, as a desirable therapeutic goal. Frankl, however, pointed out that, in the noëtic dimension, homeostasis is not a desirable condition but rather a warning sign of an existential frustration. A tensionless state in the noëtic dimension would denote complete satisfaction, that is, a lack of goals. Goals are beckoning only when conditions are *not* completely satisfying and leave room for change. When people lack the necessity to change, to create, to finish a project, to experience, or at least to brave an unchangeable fate, the necessity of continuing to live may be questioned.

Frankl spoke of a "healthy noödynamism," a field of tension between what we are and what we have the vision of becoming. Such noëtic tension stands in opposition to being in balance with oneself and the world. Balance is enormously important for all life forms, but for the human being it is not enough.

Methods

From these premises, it follows that psychotherapeutic practice cannot be effective with logotherapy alone, but neither can it be effective without logotherapy.

During the past six years I have treated and kept records of 300 persons with logotherapeutic methods, either exclusively or in combination with other methods. The logotherapist who keeps the noëtic dimension firmly in mind can also use reinforcements, client-oriented discussions, free associations, autogenic training, assertiveness training, and other techniques. Combination treatments are helpful to clients but make scientific investigations difficult because it is not always clear which method(s) in the combination may have been instrumental in reaching the therapy goal.

Nevertheless, I can present some data from my statistical evidence covering four basic logotherapeutic techniques:

Modulation of attitudes: 110 clients (37%)
Paradoxical intention: 91 clients (30%)
Dereflection: 60 clients (20%)
Suggestive technique: 39 clients (13%)

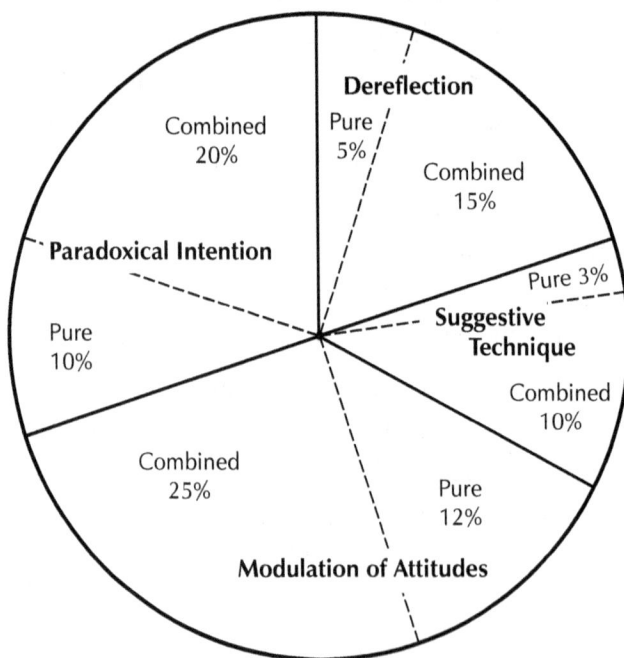

Figure 4: Logotherapeutic methods used on 300 clients

In each of the four techniques I divided my cases in two groups: application in pure form, and application in combination with other methods as depicted in Figure 4.

To judge the success of each method three criteria were considered:

a) Degree of success: 1–very good; 2–good; 3–medium; 4–poor.

b) Time to reach the therapy goal (in weeks).

c) Recidivism: number of clients and average time before further treatment (in weeks).

Modulation of attitudes

Of the 300 clients under consideration, 110 were treated by modulation of negative, unhealthy, or reductionist attitudes into attitudes that opened the clients' readiness to see or at least to search for meaning.

Results with modulation of attitudes were good to very good, were achieved within three to five weeks, and showed a varying degree of recidivism. Combination with other methods was more successful for securing lasting effects, as shown in Table 2.

Application	Number of clients	Degrees of success	Weeks to reach therapy goals	Recidivism	
				Number of clients	After # of weeks
Pure	36	2.1	3.3	9	18
Combined	74	1.4	4.8	15	41

Table 2: Results of the application of modulation of attitudes

Paradoxical intention

Paradoxical intention was applied to 91 of the 300 clients—30 in pure form, and 61 in combination with other methods. Paradoxical intention was successfully applied in combination with autogenic training, progressive relaxation, medication, assertiveness training, and raising self-esteem.

Paradoxical intention reached the therapy goal well, quickly, and with lasting results. No client treated with paradoxical intention in combination with other methods (usually autogenic training) suffered a relapse, as can be seen in Table 3 (next page).

Application	Number of clients	Degrees of success	Weeks to reach therapy goals	Recidivism	
				Number of clients	After # of weeks
Pure	30	2.5	4	6	67
Combined	61	1.3	8	None	None

Table 3: Results of the application of paradoxical intention

Dereflection

Dereflection was used on 60 clients: 15 in pure form, and 45 in combination with other methods, often with goal-oriented reinforcement.

The degree of success was good, but length of treatment and inclination to recidivism was greater than with paradoxical intention, as can be seen in Table 4.

Application	Number of clients	Degrees of success	Weeks to reach therapy goals	Recidivism	
				Number of clients	After # of weeks
Pure	15	2.8	10	6	19
Combined	45	1.6	13	9	33

Table 4: Results of the application of dereflection

Suggestive technique

The suggestive technique operates in the psychological dimension of the human being but opens the way to activating the resources of the spirit. Because the forces of the human spirit are identical with the will of a person, I have designed a logotherapeutic *suggestive training of the will* that can be used when individuals are not able to cooperate actively with a therapy because they lack insight or are too old, too young, too sick, or too upset to make decisions and act upon them.

The suggestion must not address the goal of therapy; that is what the clients will have to reach by themselves. Their freedom to decide must remain theirs; only the obstacles that may block that freedom can be removed by the suggestive technique. The suggestive training of the will, therefore, may be formulated along these lines:

I am not the helpless victim of my drives and my emotions. I
have a free will, and I am going to strengthen my will, to reshape
my life in a new way, in a direction of goals that are meaningful
to me, in a direction of ideals which are honestly mine. I feel this
inner will; it awakens in me, becomes stronger and stronger, it
gives me strength to persist. I shall master my life in spite of all
the drawbacks. The greater the difficulties, the greater will be my
strength.

In my practice, the suggestive technique was used on 39 individuals—9
in pure form and 30 in combination with other methods (mostly assertiveness training).

The suggestive technique showed good-to-medium therapy success
in a relatively short time; however, the time needed was longer than with
the other methods, and with a medium tendency to recidivism. It must
be remembered that the technique was used on clients with the greatest
resistance to therapy, as shown in Table 5.

| Application | Number of clients | Degrees of success | Weeks to reach therapy goals | Recidivism | |
				Number of clients	After # of weeks
Pure	9	2.4	9	6	11
Combined	30	2.9	15	12	8

Table 5: Results of the application of the suggestive technique

Don't look for yourself,
you won't find yourself.
In endless analyses
you become a distortion
in the abyss of dreams.

Look for beautiful experiences,
surrender to them.
In timeless moments
of bliss you will get glimpses
of your identity.

Look for meaningful tasks
and devote yourself to them.
In many building blocks
of fulfillment you will discover
your creativity.

Look for the courageous bearing
of the unavoidable.
In silent, bitter hours
of suffering you will grow
to your potential greatness.

Don't look for yourslf,
you won't find yourself.
You will be shaped
   in unselfish love,
      unselfish deeds,
         unselfish suffering.

                    Elisabeth Lukas

CHAPTER 22

Counseling Tactics and Personality Structure

The basic principles of logotherapy are helpful guidelines for the counselor to find the proper counseling tactics for clients with various personality structures as they come across to the counselor even in the early stages of the counseling. This article discusses 10 personality structures frequently encountered by the counselor and suggests a general counseling approach for each. Frankl called for a) individualizing the counseling process from client to client, and b) improvising it from moment to moment. The remainder of this chapter is divided into two sections, corresponding to this delineation.

To individualize the counseling process means to respond to the uniqueness of the client, though not at the price of violating basic logotherapeutic principles. The 10 personality "types," mere samples of what the counselor may face, point out two factors to be considered: The client's personality structure that emerges during the sessions, and the basic principles of logotherapy. Clients must not be treated in a way that will humiliate, offend, cause pain, or make them insecure, but neither must they be comforted, supported, or made to cooperate by means contrary to the principles of logotherapy. The therapy plan must not be overdemanding, distressing, or unacceptable to the client, even if it contains the best methods; neither must the plan be questionable in its methods, even if the client likes it.

To improvise does not mean to apply therapy spontaneously or on a whim, but to plan carefully according to the client's personality and the requirements of the presenting problems. If individualization means meeting the patients on a solid path, then improvisation means building bridges that can be safely crossed as the need arises.

A. INDIVIDUALIZING FROM CLIENT TO CLIENT

Counselors know that they must approach clients in different ways even if the problems are the same and the symptoms are similar.

The first counseling session offers valuable indications for the subsequent counseling procedure. It clearly reveals the clients' attitudes toward the counselor, what they expect and hope for, in what form they look for—and demand—help, and how they see the role of the counselor. The first contact offers the opportunity to appraise the personality structure of the clients, exactly because both parties are still strangers. The skillful counselor therefore will focus attention, during the first session, not so much on analyzing the problems presented, which in their totality cannot be grasped so quickly anyway—but rather on preparing the counseling tactics that will be most suitable to the personality structure of the clients.

IMPRESSIONS OF CLIENT ON COUNSELOR	**APPROPRIATE RESPONSE OF COUNSELOR**
(Expression of client's personality structure)	*(Expression of counselor's tactics)*

1. The Insecure

Such clients say little, are soft-spoken, incoherent. They cannot express clearly what they want, avoid eye contact, may smoke continuously or move their hands nervously. They appear shy, inhibited, unstable, as if ready to jump up or leave. They find it difficult to trust, to feel hopeful. They are fixated on their problems yet can hardly verbalize them. Often they have been "sent" by someone else and find it hard to bring themselves to come in for help.	The counselor should not make the mistake of underestimating the client's intelligence because of their dysfunctional behavior. They can be helped by gently guiding them toward topics in which they feel secure. It is important to inquire about positive aspects of their lives and to take them seriously. The real problems should be touched only marginally to avoid the danger of hyperreflection. It is mandatory to first gain the trust of the clients; otherwise, it is impossible to reduce their difficulties.

Basic Principle: By gaining trust in another person the trust in life can be renewed.

2. The Arrogant

The clients know exactly what they want, have definite concerns, and want to "use" the counselor to help them deal with their concerns. They expect the counselor to behave to their liking, to which they feel entitled because they pay for the treatment. If the counselor does not comply with their wishes, they know they can find another one. Occasionally this attitude leads to some form of blackmail; quick solutions are expected, failures are blamed on the counselor's incompetence. Money often is no object.

The counselor must not allow being placed in the role of a "mechanic" who is doing a repair job, or the clients are reduced to broken-down machines to be fixed.

Further, it must be made clear to such clients that the rate of the fees does not determine the counseling effort—professional ethics demand that counselors help regardless of client status. Thirdly, and most importantly, the counselor must make clear that the therapy goal does not entirely depend on clients' wishes. What can be achieved and what should be achieved are two different things: the first depends on what is technically possible; the second on the existential needs of the clients.

Basic Principle: The highest criterion of the treatment is its meaning potential.

3. The Pessimistic

Such clients emphasize up front that they expect little from the counseling. They only came to make sure they have "tried everything," but they don't believe in any success or even in the possibility that their problems can be solved. That's why they hardly find it worthwhile to talk about their problems. They give the impression of being resigned rather than hostile, but make it clear that they are not ready to share any optimism. Occasionally, they directly announce their lack of willingness to cooperate: The counselor can go ahead and try but they themselves don't see much sense in any counseling suggestions.

The counselor must not become provoked by this show of pessimism because it often hides fear or immaturity. Neither must the counselor accept the pessimism because this will fortify it. The clients have to be told quietly and factually that it is up to them to change their situation, and that the counselor can only function as a temporary crutch if the clients want to learn to walk on their own legs. If the clients don't want to do this, the crutch will be worthless. Therefore, it is necessary to make these individuals aware of their own responsibility without denying them the offer to help.

Basic Principle: Only the awareness of self-responsibility makes the acceptance of outside help meaningful.

4. The Flighty

These individuals have serious problems that they minimize; they refuse to pay too much attention to them. They display an unjustified optimism: Everything will come out all right, even if they won't follow the therapeutic advice that is offered. They are aware, however, that their attitude holds a danger to their health and may harm other people (as, for instance, driving under the influence of alcohol) and that they ought to take their problems seriously. But they find it uncomfortable to talk about these problems and to work on themselves, and so they escape into unrealistic hopes. Illusions blur their awareness of reality, which alone could motivate them to act.

To destroy illusions and bring out negative facts are among the counselor's most disagreeable tasks. Therefore, it is imperative in each case to consider carefully whether such actions are really necessary and, if so, to what extent. Sometimes, however, addressing problems head on is required to prevent more serious damage, as, for instance, commitment in an institution, separation from another person, or abandonment of educational pursuits. Though proceeding forward to deal with the problems directly will cause great pain to the clients, the counselor must proceed like a surgeon and make the painful cut but always in hopes of restoring health. Even if the prognosis is poor, the counselor must be guided only by the consideration of what the negative consequences might be if *no* therapy is provided, never by those that might occur *in spite of* the therapy.

Basic Principle: One can live with disappointment, pain, and abandonment but not with hopelessness.

5. The Depressed

These individuals have suffered a severe loss and cannot get over it. They constantly talk about it, weep, are in despair. They are not receptive to counseling efforts and shut themselves off from the world because they are submerged in their pain. Talking about the pain is helpful but also compounds the despair. Often this situation illustrates the collapse of a "pyramidal value hierarchy," the tendency to idolize one value, which now has been lost.

Every form of reaction which brings excessive depressive symptoms calls for caution, and the counselor will do well to seek the assistance of a physician. To play down the loss ("it's not the end of the world," etc.) is of little help, and may be resented by clients who feel misunderstood. For this reason, it is advisable for the counselor to accept clients' feelings of loss but at the same time to help them search for a meaning behind the situation. To accomplish this, clients must learn to listen. Their continuous laments must be gently but firmly interrupted, and every effort must be made to slowly gain the clients' attention and to begin to focus on more healthy possibilities in the present and future.

Basic Principle: To relieve pain by talking and weeping is beneficial but only up to a point.

6. The Aggressive

From the beginning, these clients display irritated and emotional reactions, perhaps even becoming outraged. Their voices rise, their faces become red, their breath goes fast, perspiration shows on their foreheads. They become agitated about trifles, aggressive toward the counselor, and irritated toward others. They get hung up on irrelevancies and angrily defend their "rights" or points of view. Their aggression may be hidden and burst forth only at certain moments of the session, but when it happens it is out of all proportion. Contradiction incites their emotional behavior, but so also does sensitive understanding. They may accompany their words and gestures with a sudden outburst of tears.

The counselor of such temperamental, emotional persons must not wait too long to get on top of the situation, or there will be the risk of a "hysterical attack." It is good to point out, as soon as this tendency is noticed, that a modicum of regard and politeness is required to discuss the problem. Clients are invited to sit down comfortably and breathe quietly before they state their case slowly and rationally. If a topic is so laden with emotions for them that a reasonable discussion is impossible, the counselor should not hesitate to break off the discussion of the topic and postpone it for another time. Relaxation exercises may be offered, but tears should not be allowed to have any effect.

Basic Principle: Where a modicum of self-discipline is lacking, the forces of the spirit are powerless.

7. The Conformist ("Dependent on Authority")

These individuals are indecisive about what they really want, they are looking for help in their decisions from "the expert." They fret because they want to do everything right and do not have the courage for spontaneous decisions. They often show a blind belief in authority: Only the expert can tell them what to do. These clients may have gathered pedantically what could weigh for or against a certain decision, and the list is presented to the counselor for the pronouncement of wise judgment. Without expressing it in so many words, the clients' behavior in many cases indicates the wish that the counselor take over the decision making—as the truly "competent" person.

The counselor must not presume to be able to always make the right decision, especially not on the basis of a handful of information. But neither must the counselor, on principle, refuse to give an answer to a question. The counselor must balance how far the clients can be trusted to reach meaningful decisions by themselves, and where they need direction to prevent them from getting into unfortunate situations. This weighing must not show, but the clients have to be made aware of some higher goals so they may distinguish essentials from nonessentials. A strengthening of the clients' ability to realize these distinctions may make direction-giving superfluous.

Basic Principle: The goal decides the means to reach it.

8. The Intellectual

Individuals who have this trait seem unnaturally aloof and composed, perhaps also unemotional and inwardly rigid. They analyze their problems and carefully interpret their situations, without revealing any inner feelings or concern. One is tempted to tag such clients as "typical intellectuals" who wish the counseling for theoretical discussions to show off their minds, perhaps to discuss merely for the sake of discussing. The entire area of the emotions is disregarded, even treated with irony; they may be crowded out by philosophical or political ideas or explained away by rational arguments. Arguments from others are hardly accepted.

The counselor must be careful not to be drawn into verbal shadow boxing that does not connect with therapeutic gains. The counseling session does not serve primarily to debate about various opinions and discuss theories. The sessions should aim at a gradual deintellectualization of the clients, at the expansion of their experiential sphere which may stimulate them to resonate to their emotions. Because there is the danger of "talking a problem to death," demonstrations and practical activities are helpful to stimulate the clients' "prereflective" understanding of themselves and their values, e.g., a shared walk through the woods, a common visit to a hospital, or similar events where impressions and experiences are stronger than words.

Basic Principle: Emotions can be more sensitive than the mind can be sensible.

9. The Dependent

These individuals present themselves in the best light and blame everyone else as responsible for their problems. Sometimes the past or mistakes by others also serve as excuses for present difficulties. These clients look to the counselor for the confirmation that they are not at fault and they could not have acted differently than they did. They want a sympathetic counselor who will help them piece together a chain of outside causes that would completely explain their present failures. Advice that aims to draw their attention to their own freedom to act is shot down or ignored, and interpreted as "misunderstanding."

The counselor's task is to confront such determinism (which they tend to corroborate with supportive pseudoinformation) in order to revive the client's freedom of will and their defiant power of the spirit, which appear to be blocked. To this end, the counselor must strictly refuse to accept the arguments of the clients and pronounce an unassailable "No." Together with the clients' "guilt," the counselor also restores their dignity; along with responsibility the inherent spiritual freedom is reinstated. The initial shock of the therapeutic harshness is softened by the acceptance of the clients as human beings, gifted with reason and the capacity for decisions, who may not always be understood but are always taken as genuine.

Basic Principle: To possess freedom of spirit is to be free from the enslavement by any conditions.

10. The Lethargic

These clients are empty and burned out—they face the counselor with indifference. They answer questions with a "yes" or "no." Nothing means anything to them. Hardly a topic can be found that lures them from their reserve. Everything bores them, passes them by, and all efforts by the counselor bring only a yawn. In severe cases, there is a danger of suicide. Often the damage is done by neglect but affluence may be responsible: Leisure time is spent in boredom, with no motivation to reach any goal. The chronic condition of the clients is absolute listlessness.

Whenever such a noögenic difficulty exists, the counselor must be aware that the existential foundations of the clients have become shaky, and there is danger to life, even if only a danger to the life of the spiritual dimension. For this reason, the counselor must carefully investigate the clients' living conditions, to find out whether a change in these conditions might revive the impulses for motivations. Extreme caution is required. For example, to make such clients financially secure may be harmful because this would make unnecessary any efforts on their part to consciously do something about their situation. It may be helpful to include family members in the counseling process, and with their help find modest short-range goals that the clients can—or must—accept.

Basic Principle: Into the existential vacuum may enter life-threatening forms of sickness.

B. IMPROVISING FROM MOMENT TO MOMENT

The clients' personality structure influences not only the counselor's proper response to the individual client but also the most effective therapy plan that can be found for specific problems.

In the first part of this article I have illustrated the proper response of the counselor in one single situation—the initial counseling session. I will now illustrate for the same ten personality structures how the therapy plan will differ according to the clients' reactions to their problems—this time in relation to one single symptom. To exclude possible complex interrelations with other symptoms and even more complex feedback effects on the total picture of the clients' sickness, I have chosen a simple, one-dimensional symptom—an isolated weakness of concentration.

REACTION OF CLIENTS TO SYMPTOM	THE THERAPY PLAN
(Expression of client's personality structure)	*(Expression of counselor's tactics)*

1 . The Insecure

Because of their inability to concentrate, these individuals feel even more insecure; they hardly dare to meet others and have little confidence to take on new tasks. They are withdrawn, speak softly, if at all. Their thoughts wander. Because of their insecurity, they give the impression of being confused, overly shy, sometimes look ridiculous, and may be ignored by others or considered not "all there." Thus, they become increasingly isolated and introverted. Others may think of them as "odd." Sometimes they lose contact with their surroundings altogether and avoid all communication with others.

Because these individuals need to gain more confidence in their interaction with others, the first step toward this goal can be achieved in the client-counselor dialogue. Using a mild form of paradoxical intention, the counselor may tell briefly about an interesting event and ask the clients not to concentrate on the story so they will have no recollection of it. Asked about it later, the clients presumably will admit to remember some details of the story. Then a switch of roles is suggested: The client tells about an event and the counselor listens. By telling the story, the clients have to concentrate and thus train their capacity of concentration while reducing their anxiety about their inability to concentrate.

Basic Principle: Fear brings about that which is feared.

2. The Arrogant

Clients are eager to overcome their weakness of concentration because they feel it prevents them from being successful in their profession or in other areas of life. They would like to get hold of a box of "concentration pills" which would solve their problem quickly and once and for all Because such pills do not exist, they are willing to go through a training program, on condition that a speedy improvement is guaranteed. They are convinced the problem can be solved if only the right remedy is found, and they are determined to succeed in overcoming their malady. Any suggestion that the weakness may have physical causes, such as old age, are hardly acknowledged.

Because clients want to force something, there is the acute danger they will not reach their goal even if they spend a lot of money in trying. The counselor must evaluate the possibility that "better concentration" is not as important a goal as, for instance, the achievement of inner peace and a feeling of fulfillment. It may be necessary to explain to these individuals that a hectic pursuit of success is counterproductive because success must not be directly pursued but must *ensue*. In the course of counseling, clients should be helped to see more clearly the goals for which it would be meaningful to strengthen their concentration, and to realize that efforts in a different direction perhaps may be more rewarding.

Basic Principle: Success and happiness are mere side effects of the pursuit of a meaningful goal.

3. The Pessimistic

These individuals see the future course of their lives as predetermined: The weakness of concentration is only the beginning, then other troubles will come, more failures, and it will all end with a mental breakdown or other serious difficulties. They always have had bad luck, and it is obviously their fate to age, become decrepit and forgetful before their time. In short, it won't be long before they won't be able to function at all. They don't believe they can be helped. In fact, they are sure that modern pharmaceuticals only make people sicker; in general, these are hopeless times in which we live.

As soon as the clients go from a negative prognosis of their own symptoms to general pessimistic observations on the state of the world, their train of thought must be stopped; they must be led back to the essentials of their case. It makes little sense to work on their specific symptom—the inability to concentrate—because even if this symptom is improved, they would find other negative aspects of their lives which will make them think of other dark scenarios. This type of individual can be greatly helped by a dereflection group that intentionally accentuates the positive and prevents the participants from wallowing only in the negative aspects of their lives. A dereflection group will regenerate their perception of values so they can see and accept also the good and beautiful around them.[1]

Basic Principle: The positive is in us, or nowhere at all.

---

1   For a detailed description of a dereflection group, see chapter 11 in Lukas, E. (2020). *Understanding Man's Search for Meaning*, pp. 117-134: "A person's admission into self-responsibility: Reducing the relapse rate in psychotherapy." See also chapter 6 in Lukas, E. (2015). *Meaning in Suffering*, pp. 87–99: "The will to joy as a health resource". –Ed.

4. The Flighty

Individuals with this personality trait have serious difficulties with concentration, which could be the result of considerable stress or the onset of a sickness. But they don't want to think about that and feel they can handle the difficulty without outside help. But they make serious mistakes in their work or their lives in general, with consequences that cannot easily be corrected. They may carelessly jaywalk in heavy traffic or forget important appointments. Their family and friends urge them to seek professional help, and so they finally come to see a counselor.

If no physician has been consulted, the counselor needs to ensure that the presenting problems have no organic causes that could be treated medically. Even so, it is useful to convince these individuals of the desirability of a healthy lifestyle— sensible nutrition, relaxation, and exercise. A restful vacation may prevent a worsening of the condition. After such discussions, a training program to improve concentration may be started, aimed at getting them to balance stress and leisure, strain and relaxation.

Basic Principle: All three human dimensions are inextricably interrelated and cannot be separated, even in therapy.

5. The Depressed

These clients have experienced an event that for them was tragic and which has not been worked through. They feel that they will never be able to forget it. Since that event, much has changed in their lives, primarily that they don't see much meaning in life in what is going on around them; their thoughts are still focused on the loss and the circumstances that have led up to it. For these clients, difficulties of concentration are closely linked with their attitude, the result of their lack of interest in anything not connected with that event, that is, anything lying outside their one-sided value orientation.

These symptoms are clearly the result of unavoidable suffering, so clients' attitudes to this suffering must be placed at the center of the counseling effort. A modulation of attitudes can help individuals to bear the suffering and to overcome the difficulties in concentration. When such clients talk about their suffering, attention can be focused on the fact that they are giving attention to what they are saying, thus the counseling can begin with such a conversation. The counselor has the opportunity to lead clients to see possibilities of finding a meaningful interpretation of their suffering. Only then can the attempt be made to expand their personal value orientation, and this will automatically lead to an intensified concentration on the various value contents contemplated.

Basic Principle: Every suffering has its meaning.

6. The Aggressive

Clients are terribly angry at themselves for being confused and forgetful. Every little thing that slips their minds upsets them, and they may vent their anger on others who happen to be around. The rage about these mishaps destroys the positive possibilities of their lives and prevents successes which they otherwise may have had. Sometimes they develop a self-hate which spills over onto their families and makes life miserable for everyone concerned.

Because these clients, generally speaking, do not show enough of a sense of humor for paradoxical intention, it is often better to begin with simple, calming formulations (e.g., self-suggestions and physical means, such as relaxation and breathing exercises) that enable them to regain self-control and distance from their problems. Next, a suggestive training of the will can be started. This shifts the focus from uncontrolled emotion to factual cognition: Their thinking thereby regains dominance over their feelings. On this level, clients can handle their weaknesses more effectively.

Basic Principle: One does not have to take every nonsense from one's temperament.

7. The Conformist ("Dependent on Authority")

For some time, clients have observed certain difficulties in grasping and remembering new ideas, and are uncertain what to do. They believe that an expert will see the full significance of their symptoms. Some clients will read books on the subject, which only further confuses them. They begin to observe themselves and soon notice a worsening of their difficulties, which sends them to the counselor in a panic. They ask the expert to "uncover" the causes of the problem and the "unconscious forces" behind them.

The expert can use the clients' faith in authority by explaining to them the dangerous mechanism of hyperreflection, and by exhorting them not to observe themselves or read about their symptoms on the Internet. They are told that the anxious recording of the symptoms is counterproductive. On the other hand, a carefully targeted dereflection—a concentration on the clients' surroundings—is useful in a twofold way: It counters the existing hyperreflection, strengthens the ability of concentration, and restores the self-confidence of the clients.

Basic Principle: By encouraging self-transcendence ego weakness can be transformed into ego strength.

8. The Intellectual

These clients have their own hypotheses about their problems. They tell the counselor exactly how the symptoms originated and what their effects are. This is all described in sober and correct terms. In no way do the clients indicate that the symptoms cause them suffering, they wish to discuss the concentration problems on principle and factually, and seek the expert opinion to check their own theories with those of the counselor. Sometimes they approach their goal obliquely, pretending to have a friend who suffers from these same symptoms and asking how they best can help that fictitious friend. They are inclined to see their difficulty as a problem of our age or our society, the result of an deteriorating civilization.

In general, it may be helpful to determine the extent to which the clients are capable of any deeper experiences and if so, of what kind. If they are found to be incapable of such experiences, it can be assumed that they are cut off from an entire dimension by cognitive blocks. Instead of exploring the origins of these inhibitions, the counselor can help them to revive the experiential dimension by motivating them to fill their leisure with creative activities that will stimulate their emotional responses. Experiences in art and nature, the practice of positive meditation, and opening them to significant encounters may set in motion a chain of reactions that will sharpen their capacity for concentration and stimulate their emotional responses.

Basic Principle: Finding meaning in the noëtic dimension is irrevocably tied to the capacity for emotional experiences.

9. The Dependent

These clients admit that recently they have had trouble concentrating but they blame it on the behavior of other persons, such as loud music from a child's room or impossible working conditions. They see themselves as "victims," facing an inconsiderate world, with little chance to be masters of their fate and influence their lives. Questions as to whether they have to stand for the noise of their children or whether they have ever thought of changing their working place only draws a resigned shaking of their heads.

The clients must be challenged to resistance, not so much against the stressful environment but against their own resignation. They have to be made to see that they play their part, that they are coresponsible for their difficulties, and that it is they themselves who can bring about a change. In the course of the counseling sessions it will probably turn out that the environment is less to blame than they have thought, and their resistance can then be converted into a healthy defiant power of the human spirit against their own symptoms. Thus, the difficulty is mitigated through an increasing strengthening of the clients' capacity for self-distancing.

Basic Principle: Only a healthy resistance can overcome an unhealthy dependence.

10. The Lethargic

These clients hardly talk about their symptoms; rather, they demonstrate them by being inattentive, confused, unfocused. The words of the counselor pass them by; there is no reaction and their scarce responses tend to be off topic. Their apathy stops everything; concrete suggestions lead nowhere. There is no motivation to do anything about their concentration. Sometimes a trace of defiance shows in the form of a secret smile about the counselor's efforts which are so utterly boring—what is the use of it all? To concentrate well seems just as pointless as to concentrate badly.

Despite the clients' lethargy, there certainly must be something that is important to them, something to which they are not completely indifferent. Perhaps it is a way of life that feels comfortable, a certain place they like, or contact with a person who means something to them. That would be a starting point to help clients move from a readiness to make a minimum effort to the attainment of a desired condition of human contact: They must make an effort to concentrate in order to come closer to their goal. In case they are completely without anything that seems worthy of effort, a sudden change of environment and the challenge of a new task may bring about an inner change; for instance, being sent to help in a disaster area.

Basic Principle: If you consider your life without meaning, you do not see the tasks life has in store for you.

There are some
who live by the principle:
"Everything or nothing."
A sudden suffering
overcomes them
and there remains "nothing."

There are others
who turn up their noses:
"Everything is nothing."
A sudden fortune comes
and goes,
and there remains "nothing."

There are still others
who can find "something"
in everything.
Come suffering or fortune,
they lose "nothing."

Elisabeth Lukas

CHAPTER 23

Logotherapy on Hysteria

Hysteria is among the great challenges to the therapist. Unfortunately, it has become a pejorative term. In Freud's time, its symptomatology was reported widely; much less so later, though it made a temporary comeback in the latter part of the 20th century.[1]

Those who suffer from symptoms of hysteria tend to be fascinated by negatives and to resist anything positive. This means that for the patient a cure is not necessarily the goal of therapy. Often patients participate in therapy until the goal is in sight, and then suddenly start subverting the goal. The therapist may help the client resolve numerous problems, but when the therapist says, "Now we don't need any appointments for a while, you are able to be on your own," such clients tend to respond, "If you don't give me an appointment soon, I'll have a relapse." Instead of being glad of

---

1 [The word *hysteria* comes from the Greek root *hystera,* which means "womb"; the word originated in the early part of the 19th century and was derived from the idea that only women suffer from these symptoms, which were thought to be caused by uterine disturbances. "Hysteria" was used as a term to define a psychological disorder until as recently as 1980, when the term was removed from the 3rd edition of the *Diagnostic and Statistical Manual of Mental Disorders.* Today, these symptoms are instead thought to be related to dissociative and somatoform disorders. Even "neurosis" and "psychosis" are no longer in common use. Lukas suggested that terminology such as this should be updated by referring to the origin, or genesis of disorders, as in *somatogenic* or *psychogenic.* See Lukas, E. (2016). "The Pathogenesis of Mental Disorders: An Update of Logotherapy" in Batthyány, A., Ed. *Logotherapy and Existential Analysis: Proceedings of the Viktor Frankl Institute Vienna.* Switzerland: Springer. –Ed.]

having retained stability, they are willing to sacrifice it in order to retain the therapist's attention. Rather than thanking the therapist, these clients are inclined to use blackmail to continue therapy.

Frankl listed three characteristics of such individuals:

- *Lack of authenticity.* Individuals with symptoms of hysteria lack authentic inner experiences such as genuine joy, genuine love, genuine grief. Everything is a stage setting, even their illness. As a result, they crave experiences of any kind; even negative experiences are better than none.

- *Pathological self-centeredness (narcissism).* These individuals crave attention at any price, even if it ultimately hurts them. They constantly draw attention to themselves and punish others who neglect to pay adequate attention to them.

- *Manipulative thinking/behavior.* Their behavior is calculated to meet their own desires. They are rarely interested in a given issue as such, but have ulterior motives.

A basic characteristic of hysteria is that sufferers do not self-transcend. Instead, they demand the attention of others at any price, even if that is totally unrealistic.

Individuals with this cluster of symptoms usually use them to manipulate others into behaving contrary to their own convictions. This meets the patients' needs but is also the cause for their extreme unpopularity. People tend to avoid them and, as a result, such clients feel isolated and unhappy. To draw attention and sympathy from others, they may even harm themselves. The ultimate result is a vicious circle—they receive less and less sympathy while they continually escalate their behavior

The basis for hysteria is not only character disposition, but also childhood experiences. Usually, individuals with these symptoms have been either neglected or overindulged as children; both have the same result. Neglected children have to sacrifice much while they are small; they no longer want to do that once they grow up. Overindulged children, on the other hand, never learn to make sacrifices, so they remain ignorant in this aspect, even as adults. This explains why hysteria was so widespread in Freud's time—there were many neglected children. It also explains why hysteria is important today—there are many overindulged children.

Attitude modulation

The treatment of hysteria requires a re-education of the total person. Patients must be motivated by the therapist to give up their hysterical behavior. This is possible only through a number of attitude modulations.

Attitude modulation aims at changing a person's negative attitude into a positive, in circumstances that are either unchangeable or can be changed only through a different attitude. It is likely that current circumstances present meaning possibilities that have gone unnoticed. Every attitude modulation aims at a healthier, better, more ethically valuable, or more positive attitude. The attitude "I can't do anything right, I'm a total failure" is unhealthy. A healthy attitude opposes anything destructive, derogative, and paralyzing; it offers a strong protection against psychological illnesses and fosters a strong ability to bear suffering in crisis situations. A positive attitude is in harmony with one's own conscience.

Two examples:

A mother suffered for many years from anorexia and poor eating habits. When she was finally cured, she was not satisfied that her eating habits were normalized. She worried that her small daughter might develop the same symptoms. Because it was risky to burden the daughter with her mother's negative expectations, an attitude modulation was conducted with her mother. She was advised: "Don't keep observing your daughter for symptoms. That could only interfere with her healthy development. Rather, work on yourself so one day you can say to yourself: I don't mind her following my example." The mother was deeply impressed by the thought that, even now, she could be an example for her daughter. It motivated her to give up her exaggerated anxiety about her daughter. She reconsidered her own behavior as well and began to change in a positive direction.

The second example concerns an elderly woman who was to go to a special clinic for a minor operation. Two years previously, her husband died

in the same clinic after severe suffering. Because of this painful association, she refused to go to that clinic, the only one in that area equipped to
perform her operation.

It was gently suggested that a return to the place where she parted
from her husband might present an opportunity to come to terms with the
parting. It might lead to a feeling of thankfulness that she had been able to
be with her beloved partner to the very end—to be at his side in his hour
of greatest need. The clinic could be seen as a symbol of her love for him,
a place she could enter with confidence and a clear conscience. After this
discussion, the woman no longer resisted going to the clinic.

Small sacrifices

Logotherapeutic approaches can help individuals with symptoms of
hysteria by motivating them to develop a willingness to make small sacrifices. However, these clients will become involved only if they know what
for. This "what for" will have to be explained to them: The way to great
meaning contents in life is through small sacrifices. The unintended side
effect of great meaning contents is happiness. Conversely, acquiring small
immediate gratifications is incompatible with making small sacrifices and,
as a result, great meanings remained unfulfilled and the unavoidable side
effect is unhappiness.

For example, a person who wants to study medicine must make a series
of small sacrifices, such as preparing for an exam instead of enjoying an
evening or weekend. But this individual can realize a great meaning content
through these sacrifices by becoming a physician holding a responsible
and important position. If this student does not want to make these small
sacrifices but seeks immediate gratification in dancing, skiing, and other
pleasurable activities, the great meaning content of a professional career
evaporates and may eventually lead to a humdrum, disliked job.

Heart neurosis

Sometimes hysteria takes the form of a heart neurosis. Every time the
family is happy and celebrating, a family member develops a heart condition.

The celebration is spoiled, everyone is concerned, and happiness is gone. The display of the heart condition brings immediate gratification to the family member, who has become the center of attention. The long-term consequences, however, lead to unhappiness. The children may leave the home earlier, the spouse may file for divorce. Ultimately the health of the family member displaying these symptoms may actually be affected and eventually he or she becomes progressively bitter and lonely.

Therapy should aim at uncovering this threatening catastrophe, not by way of reproach but out of genuine concern. Somehow the therapist should signal: "I like you, but not your hysteria." To differentiate between what a person *is* and what a person *has* is important in logotherapy.

What does the family member, in the heart-neurosis example, *have?* A few hours of enforced attention from the family; even that will rapidly wane. But what *is* that individual? An individual who has an illness. Nobody likes to be with this family member because everybody is afraid of the next hysterical outburst. This is the way it will be until the end of that person's life if his or her attitude does not change radically. Even after death, such a person will be remembered as the one who was shunned—*being* is forever, even if it is a *being-in-the-past*.

Therapy must focus on the person this individual could be—a loved spouse and parent, visited gladly by every family member because of their support. Is that perhaps what is deeply wanted? If this should be the case, the logotherapist can show the way. But it requires giving up melodramatics, being prepared to take the back seat once in a while, and allowing others to enjoy themselves. This way leads from *having* to *being*.

Treating hysteria

The individual who suffers from symptoms of hysteria has a talent for melodrama that can be used in a positive way. The therapist can outline a new role and challenge the patient to play-act this character. In the case of the family member with the heart neurosis, the role of a selfless, lovable parent might be tried. It is possible to wonder what good is it if such a person only *plays* a better character; it is not genuine. This is not the case with hysteria, in which transition between the conscious and unconscious, between the genuine and false, are fluid. In fact, one of the greatest dangers with these individuals is that they identify so strongly with their initial, faked, unhealthy character that they cannot shake it off even when they want to. It is as if they have no textbook for enacting a positive character, and it is up to the therapist to provide one. The symptoms may take on a life of their own. In our example, it is possible that the family member actually develops an arrhythmia of her heart, whether wanted or not. If for those who suffer from hysteria the transitions between the unconscious and conscious are so fluid, why shouldn't they be able to identify with a positive role, when in the long run it gains so much more attention than the negative one? At some point, the person must be made aware of this possibility.

It is, however, not the therapist's job to play along with the hysteric's melodramatics. They love long-term therapy because it provides them with what they need: They are the center of attention with an understanding listener. If they have alienated the rest of the world, the therapist may be the last person who cares to listen. In exchange, they pay not only with money but with stories, whatever the therapist wants to hear—from terrible childhood experiences to wild dreams or sexual fantasies. But that does not solve any problems. If the therapist determines that the therapeutic arguments are not taken seriously, and the patient refuses to play a positive role or declines to make a meaningful sacrifice for the sake of realizing genuine values, or uses therapy as substitute for meaning, the therapist must end the treatment.

Therapists cannot help everyone, but they must not harm them either. Playing along with hysterical behavior is harmful. Today, sociogenic factors support this playing along. Individuals with hysteric symptoms are tempted to fill their leisure time by undergoing therapy while therapists who need clients are only too willing to provide this "leisure activity." This results in people being harmed by therapy and therapy sinking into disrepute.

It has been my experience that, with some regularity, one week before my vacation several of my clients have "attacks" and are at "death's door."

This is supposed to give me the message: "How dare you go on vacation and be unavailable to me?" They want me to know that, if I must go on vacation, at least I should go with a heavy heart and a bad conscience. Certainly, persons suffering from hysteria are emotionally disabled; they can, however, still be responsible for their actions. That is exactly what they have to learn, even if it is a slow and difficult process.

I know of a dark street
running through the soul.
Many of our thoughts
travel on it.

The street sign says: egoism,
the cobblestones are blind drives,
many of our intentions
trip over them.

On the side of the street
the guideposts point to lust and power.
Our earthly desires
follow their directions.

But at the end of the street
the travelers are stopped,
halted by the words:
Blind Alley.

Elisabeth Lukas

CHAPTER 24

Logotherapy in the Practice
of Clinical Psychology

S trictly speaking, clinical psychology is many years younger than logotherapy. The "clinical" part of psychology, that is the practical application of its theories, was until recently part of medicine; logotherapy, too, has its roots in medical science.

But psychology is not only a young science; as is fitting for youth, it is also an aggressive discipline. Practitioners press forward to gain ground, and are lucky to find the Western world in a condition where the discipline is badly needed.

Today, we are protected not only by a social net, but by something that could be called a "psychological net." We are exposed to ideas of psychology everywhere—in school, at work, in court, and in the clinic. You ask people how they did "at their psychologist," and the answers range from an embarrassed shrug to a more or less veiled expression of annoyance, and once in a while some praise. But praise is rare. The practice of clinical psychology—as a young, aggressive, and sometimes tactless discipline—is viewed with suspicion by physicians and patients alike.

For these growing pains, the older approach of logotherapy could be a motherly aid. It could advise clinical psychology because it has *knowledge* and *wisdom*. Logotherapy has knowledge in that it has pieced together a mosaic of basic anthropological understanding of human nature, which can easily be applied in individual cases. To add this knowledge to the therapeutic intervention would expand its scope, and also enrich the art of improvisation and individualization that is badly needed in clinical daily practice.

Logotherapy's wisdom is needed because every therapeutic intervention is an interpersonal encounter that must never lose sight of empathy and human dignity. Logotherapists are well aware of this fact and have developed something like "professional ethical guidelines." If such guidelines are considered, therapeutic mistakes and iatrogenic damage could be prevented, and the reputation of psychology would benefit.

The knowledge base of logotherapy

- Practitioners of logotherapy know the essence of human beings and what they are striving for, that which guides them in their search.
- Those who practice logotherapy know about arousing human spiritual resources and makes therapeutic use of these.
- Logotherapists know what keeps people going in situations of unavoidable suffering, and are able to offer support to others in their journeys.

An illustration can be drawn from a symposium of gynecologists in Munich, during which a problem was discussed extensively but no solution was found. The problem, stated simply, is that science is now in a position to foretell, with 90 percent accuracy, whether a baby will be born with defects. The physicians faced the question of how they should tell the parents about such an unfavorable prognosis. In their dilemma, they had the idea to consult with psychologists. Who but a clinical psychologist would be able to solve this problem? The symposium recommended that such advice be sought.

The attempt failed because, surprisingly, the clinical psychologists had no helpful suggestions. They hinted at some mystical connections between an unwanted child and its possible defects, and then withdrew from the problem. No general prescription was provided for talks with parents.

The psychologists said it depended on the circumstances; it was a matter of judgment. Besides, they added, this type of dilemma was beyond the competency of a clinical psychologist.

For this dilemma, logotherapy can offer its rich experiences. But logotherapists, too, will not do any *pre*scribing and rather *de*scribe what is important in such cases. And what is generally important to individuals is not so much that everything be pleasant, that everyone be healthy and have enough material things to enjoy life. All this is welcome when it happens, but it is not an absolute existential necessity. What is important is that people experience their lives as meaningful and, when the end comes, that they see they have not lived in vain.

In our case, this means: The birth of a child with disabilities does not reduce the meaning of its parents' lives; on the contrary, it offers the possibility of new tasks to fulfill. And the greater the difficulties, the more vital are those tasks. This is why parents can be told: "Whatever fate has in store for you, now you are needed more than ever. Your love is needed, your cooperation, your unconditional "yes" to the child. If you find the strength for this, fate cannot do you any harm."

The question remains how the parents will muster this strength. Here, too, logotherapy can be helpful by arousing their potential strength from the resources of the human spirit. Frankl himself, by his own example, has illustrated what the defiant power of the spirit can do. As if a mysterious spark would leap across, an example of heroism has an encouraging effect on others. The contagious heroism, in this case, is the inner attitude someone is able to take in the face of unavoidable suffering—an attitude that kindles admiration and respect in others. Logotherapy offers the method of attitude modulation that helps people confronting their fate to find a healthy and affirmative attitude.

Through Socratic dialogue, the logotherapist may be able to show the prospective parents that many families are unhappy even though their children have developed normally; conversely, many a happy family was able to integrate a handicapped child into their circle. Defects, in whatever form, are no sentence to unhappiness but a challenge to the human spirit to make the best of a situation. And in the end, the situation may turn out even better than it would have been without that challenge.

One last question remains: the question of the existential anchoring of such a positive attitude. Of course, logotherapy does not presume to compete with religion. But if we are not anchored in some faith that enables us to face the ups and downs of life, we have to face these questions through philosophy. In cases of adversity such as the medical prognosis of a defective birth, the questions that demand answers are: "Why?" or "Why me?"

Physicians or psychologists ought to have some kind of answer, and they can find it in the teachings of logotherapy. Logotherapeutic experience shows that questions borne of suffering require patience because the answers may become manifest only much later—it is only in retrospect that many things become clear that are initially hidden. The prospective parents have to be helped to see that they need time to come to a conclusion about the situation. If there is a consensus among parents of children with disabilities, it is the realization that they would not have wanted to miss having had just those children. And this, after all, is a great comfort.

The wisdom of logotherapy

This example indicates that clinical psychology needs the complementary knowledge of logotherapy. But knowledge is not enough; scientific knowledge in itself is not sufficient to save humankind, as we have learned from the atomic research in scientific laboratories. The knowledge of science must be complemented by wisdom, and this is true also for clinical psychology, whose therapeutic techniques and psychological strategies too easily propel patients into subhuman, if not inhuman, channels and plunge them deeper into illness.

What is the logotherapeutic wisdom that may have significance for clinical psychology? Not the development of new fashionable techniques but rather a consideration of the basic values and goals of all therapy. These professional ethical guidelines may be listed under the following headings:

1. Normalize, don't psychologize.

2. Encourage self-help.

3. Don't take away responsibility.

The first point admittedly sounds provocative, and yet it contains an ancient wisdom that tells us to let sleeping dogs lie, or not to solve problems that do not yet (or no longer) exist. The Socratic dialogue of logotherapy requires a high degree of caution and intuition. It should not be done in an attempt to tear open old wounds at any price so they will start bleeding again and only increase the pain. Nor should it draw attention to present failures in order to see them as excuses for future ones.

If people consider themselves to be psychologically ill, this in itself traps them in their illness; tracing the dysfunctional development only paralyzes their resistance against the disorder. Therefore, we have to be careful with hypotheses and interpretations and direct our therapeutic attention to the successes of a life, to what is positive and valuable in a human existence. Old scars, for instance, may form a strong, tear-resistant tissue which, if recognized as such, will make the organism tougher and more impregnable than before.

Even pain may have its purpose; it is a powerful warning to act, to bring about change, to straighten things out. But it is the principle of hope that results in the most effective therapy as long as it is nourished by professionally justifiable means and is not choked off. In sum: Whenever the effect of psychologizing patients is greater than the gain in stabilizing them, psychotherapy becomes iatrogenic.

The reference of "stabilization" leads to the second professional ethical guideline of logotherapy—the principle of self-help. Who or what causes a physical or psychological wound to heal? Not the physicians. They can treat it with ointments and dressings but the process of healing is accomplished by the self-healing powers of the body. Modern medicine increasingly becomes convinced that health is more likely when the natural inner immune system is supported than when an attempt is made to "drive out the devil with Beelzebub," through artificial chemical interventions.

Eventually, those in the field of clinical psychology must realize that there are not only psychological causes of illnesses, but also noëtic self-healing forces which can conquer—and even prevent—such illnesses. A wise practitioner will seek out and promote these self-healing forces so that wounds will close whose origins cannot be eliminated, regardless of how intensely the patient will brood about them. All specifically logotherapeutic methods have as their goal the promotion of self-help, and the low number of relapses seems to show that they rarely miss this goal.

The third professional ethical guideline deals with responsibility. We know that not every illness can be cured and that logotherapy is no panacea. But one thing must be prevented: The practitioner must not remove responsibility from clients—the knowledge that they are responsible for their lives. Except for phases of psychotic symptoms that lie beyond the responsibility of the individual, those afflicted with mental disorders, too, have some freedom as to how to handle their illness. They can use the illness as an excuse for all sorts of things, or as a means to manipulate others. They can make it easy on themselves by claiming their parents made mistakes or that others have failed them. Especially the individual with neurotic symptoms tends in that direction.

This is the place where psychotherapeutic wisdom comes into play to challenge patients to act with responsibility within the limits of their area of freedom rather than to support their "declarations of dependence." Human beings are as dependent as they believe themselves to be, and similarly as free as they are willing to rise above their fate—that is the guideline that shows the way out of the neurotic trap.

Where there is freedom there is also responsibility, and where life is worthy of being called human, it must be directed toward a meaning that is to be fulfilled. The task of psychotherapy is not to intensify the intense self-observation and self-pity of individuals or to create a new dependency on therapy, but to help them restore their responsibility and human dignity and to become aware of why and to what end they want to get well. Psychotherapy is not a substitute for meaning!

These are the guidelines that the practice of logotherapy can offer to those in clinical psychology—not to instruct or patronize, but to help this young and promising discipline gain and earn the trust of its patients.

Depressions are clouds
darkening the day.
That's why they should be seen
as clouds.

Simply let them pass
knowing that above them,
undiminished, shines the sun
on the meaning horizon of life.

Elisabeth Lukas

www.ingramcontent.com/pod-product-compliance
Lightning Source LLC
Chambersburg PA
CBHW052134270326
41930CB00012B/2879